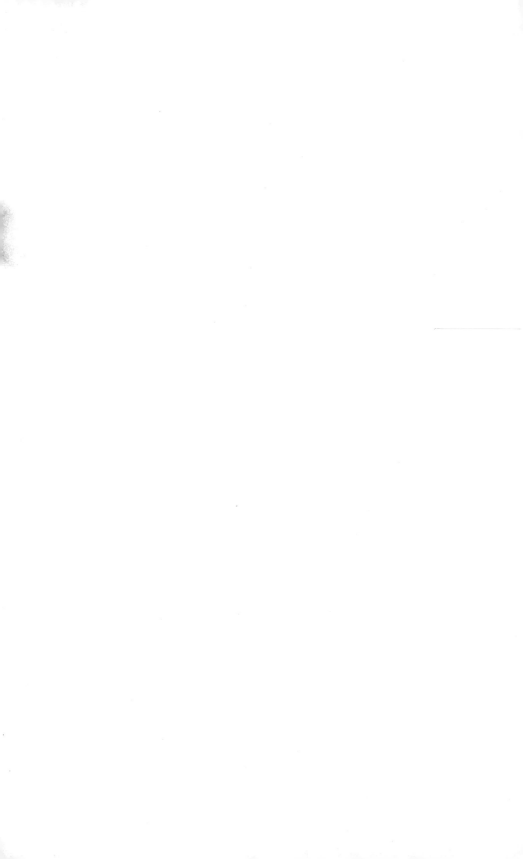

The Health Benefits of Dog Walking for People and Pets

New Directions in the Human-Animal Bond
Alan M. Beck, series editor

The Health Benefits of Dog Walking for People and Pets

Evidence and Case Studies

Rebecca A. Johnson, Alan M. Beck, and Sandra McCune

Purdue University Press
West Lafayette, Indiana

Printed in the United States of America.

Library of Congress Cataloging-in-Publication Data

The health benefits of dog walking for people and pets : evidence and case studies / [edited by] Rebecca A. Johnson, Alan M. Beck, Sandra McCune.
    p. cm.
 Summary: "This book provides the scientific evidence about the benefits of dog walking for both humans and dogs to manage weight"-- Provided by publisher.
 Includes bibliographical references and index.
 ISBN 978-1-55753-582-5 (hardback)
 1. Dog walking--Health aspects--Case studies. 2. Walking--Health aspects--Case studies. 3. Fitness walking--Case studies. 4. Dogs--Health--Case studies. 5. Human-animal relationships--Case studies. I. Johnson, Rebecca A., 1956- II. Beck, Alan M. III. McCune, Sandra K. IV. Title.

SF427.46.H43 2011
636.7'083--dc22

2011001723

Contents

List of Tables

List of Figures

Foreword

Given that the obesity and obesity-related disease epidemic continues to rage in the United States and in other industrialized countries, there exists a need to develop and examine innovative approaches to its reversal and to facilitate health and fitness. Dog walking, found to positively influence physical activity, was a focus of the symposium from which the compilation of papers presented in this volume emanated. The one-day symposium was embedded in the peer-reviewed 2009 18th Annual Conference of the International Society for Anthrozoology, which was held in Kansas City, Missouri. The symposium was entitled, "Research meets practice: Human-animal interaction in obesity across the lifespan." It was funded by an R-13 Conference Grant (R. Johnson, PI) from the *Eunice Kennedy Shriver* National Institute of Child Health and Human Development of the National Institutes of Health, and was cosponsored by Mars Waltham®.

Attended by over 300 registrants, the symposium consisted of plenary and peer-reviewed presentations and was devoted to information dissemination and dialogue promotion between health care professionals from such fields as nursing, medicine, veterinary medicine, social work, physical therapy, occupational therapy, and counseling. Additional participants were those working in animal-related fields such as animal rescue groups, animal shelters, and pet therapy visitation groups. A vital goal of the symposium was to foster collaborative projects in creative new directions between investigators and human-animal interaction and health care practitioners. Plenary speakers were Jacqueline Epping, Adrian Bauman, Audwin Fletcher, and Roland Thorpe. A variety of peer-reviewed papers and posters were also presented.

Samplings of these comprise this book. It is my sincere belief that enthusiasm from the symposium is conveyed in the exciting papers that you will find in the ensuing pages.

–Rebecca A. Johnson

Acknowledgments

We would like to thank Purdue University Press, especially Press Director Charles Watkinson, for recognizing dog walking as an area worthy of study and an intervention that helps both people and their dogs. We further extend our thanks to the *Eunice Kennedy Shriver* National Institute of Child Health and Human Development of the National Institutes of Health for funding the symposium in which the papers included in this volume were presented as part of the 2009 Annual Conference of the International Society for Anthrozoology held in Kansas City, Missouri. We are also grateful to Mars, Inc., which was the Principle Founding Sponsor for the overall conference. We would also like to thank all of the contributors of this volume, who shared their insights, findings, and experience as to how dog walking can be an interesting, fun, and healthy experience for all. Additionally, we gratefully acknowledge Charlotte McKenney for her considerable help with editing the documents for format and style.

List of Contributors

Adrian Bauman, Ph.D. F.A.F.P.H.M.
Sesquicentenary Professor of Public Health in Behavioral Epidemiology
    & Health Promotion
School of Public Health
Institute of Obesity Nutrition & Exercise (IONE)
Sydney University, Australia

Alan M. Beck, Sc.D.
Purdue University
School of Veterinary Medicine
West Lafayette, Indiana

Ashley M. Brown, M.P.H.
Executive Director, Kids and K-9s for Healthy Choices, Inc.
Denver, CO

Christopher G. Byers, D.V.M., D.A.C.V.E.C.C., D.A.C.V.I.M. (SAIM)
Director, Intensive Care VCA Veterinary Referral Associates
Gaithersburg, MD

Hayley E. Christian, Ph.D.
Research Assistant Professor
Centre for the Built Environment and Health
School of Population Health
The University of Western Australia
Perth, Australia

Carol M. Devine, Ph.D., R.D.
Division of Nutritional Sciences and Dept. of Biostatistics
Cornell University
Ithaca, NY

Denise A. Elliott B.V.Sc. (Hons) Ph.D. Dipl. A.C.V.I.M. Dipl. A.C.V.N.
Director of Health and Nutritional Sciences: The Americas
Royal Canin SAS
Aimargues, France

Jacqueline N. Epping, M.Ed.
Team Lead Guidelines and Recommendation (GAR)
Physical Activity and Health Branch
Division of Nutrition, Physical Activity and Obesity
Centers for Disease Control and Prevention
Atlanta, GA

Layla Esposito, Ph.D.
Health Scientist Administrator
Center for Research for Mothers and Children
Eunice Kennedy Shriver National Institute of Child Health and Human
    Development
National Institutes of Health
Rockville, MD

Tracy Farrell, Ph.D.
Program on Breast Cancer & Environmental Risk Factors
Cornell University
Ithaca, NY

Jeffrey L. Goodie, Ph.D., A.B.P.P.
LCDR, United States Public Health Service Assistant Professor of Family
    Medicine
Uniformed Services University of the Health Sciences
Bethesda, Maryland.

James A. Griffin, Ph.D.
Deputy Chief, Child Development & Behavior Branch
Center for Research for Mothers and Children

Eunice Kennedy Shriver National Institute of Child Health and Human Development
National Institutes of Health
Rockville, MD

Karyl J. Hurley, D.V.M., D.A.C.V.I.M., D.E.C.V.I.M.-C.A.
Global Scientific Affairs, WALTHAM
MARS PETCARE
McLean, VA

Rebecca A. Johnson, Ph.D., R.N., F.A.A.N.
Millsap Professor of Gerontological Nursing & Public Policy
Sinclair School of Nursing
Director, Research Center for Human Animal Interaction
College of Veterinary Medicine
University of Missouri
Columbia, MO

Grace Long, D.V.M., M.S., M.B.A.
Nestlé-Purina Pet Care Company
St. Louis, MO

Elizabeth Lund, D.V.M., M.P.H., Ph.D.
Senior Director of Research, Banfield Applied Research and Knowledge
Banfield, The Pet Hospital
Portland, OR

Rona Macniven, M.Sc., B.Sc. (Hons)
School of Public Health
University of Sydney, Australia.

Mary Maley, M.S.
Program on Breast Cancer & Environmental Risk Factors
Cornell University
Ithaca, NY

Sandra McCune V.N., B.A., Ph.D.
Program Manager,
Human-Companion Animal Bond Research Program,

WALTHAM Centre for Pet Nutrition (part of Mars, Inc)
Waltham-On-The-Wolds,
Melton Mobray,
U.K.

Charlotte A. McKenney, R.N., B.S.N.
Assistant Director
Research Center for Human Animal Interaction
University of Missouri
College of Veterinary Medicine
Columbia, MO

F. Ellen Netting, Ph.D., M.S.S.W.
Professor and Samuel S. Wurtzel Endowed Chair
Virginia Commonwealth University School of Social Work
Richmond, VA

Cara Olsen, Ed.D.
Assistant Professor of Preventive Medicine and Biostatistics
Uniformed Services University of the Health Sciences
Bethesda, MD

Mark B. Stephens, M.D., M.S., F.A.A.F.P.
CAPT MC USN
Associate Professor and Chair
Department of Family Medicine
Uniformed Services University of the Health Sciences
Bethesda, MD

Angela M. Struble, B.S.
Clinical Nutrition Program
Cornell University College of Veterinary Medicine
Ithaca, NY

Roland J. Thorpe, Jr., Ph.D.
Assistant Scientist
Hopkins Center for Health Disparities Solutions
Department of Health Policy and Management
Johns Hopkins Bloomberg School of Public Health
Baltimore, MD

Joseph J. Wakshlag, D.V.M., Ph.D.
Clinical Nutrition Program
Cornell University College of Veterinary Medicine
Ithaca, NY

Barbour S. Warren, Ph.D.
Program on Breast Cancer & Environmental Risk Factors
Cornell University
Ithaca, NY

Martin T. Wells, Ph.D.
Department of Biostatistics
Cornell University
Ithaca, NY

Cindy C. Wilson, Civ, Ph.D., C.H.E.S.
Professor & Faculty Development Director
Department of Family Medicine
Uniformed Services University of the Health Sciences
Bethesda, MD

Lisa J. Wood, Ph.D.
Research Assistant Professor,
Deputy Director
Centre for the Built Environment and Health
School of Population Health
The University of Western Australia
Perth, Australia

Kathy K. Wright, R.N., M.S.N., C.P.N.P.
Robert Wood Johnson Foundation Executive Nurse Fellow (2008-2011)
Nursing Director, Florida Department of Health Children's Medical Services,
    Ocala Area Office
Creative Director, Kids and K-9s for Healthy Choices, Inc.
Ocala, FL

Mary E. Yonemura
Internal Medicine—Critical Care Department VCA Veterinary Referral
    Associates
Gaithersburg, MD

Chapter 1

Dog walking as a new area of inquiry: An overview

Alan M. Beck

E. O. Wilson suggested that throughout most of human evolution survival favored those with an ability to hunt animals and find edible plants. This innate "hard-wiring" gave us a predisposition to pay special attention to animals and the surrounding environment. He named this "innate tendency to focus on life and lifelike processes" the biophilia hypothesis (Wilson, 1993). It is reasonable to assume part of our fascination with our pets, and our desire to be with them, stems from this inborn love of life, our biophilia.

In addition, like any social species, we are especially driven to be with our own kind. Most people feel adrift or lonely when isolated from others but find physical and emotional comfort when with family, friends, co-workers, and neighbors (Hawkley & Cacioppo, 2007; Lynch, 1977, 2000). Social support is the knowledge that we are part of a community of people who love, care, and value us (Weinick, 1998). This social support theory also reinforces our care for our pets, as most people incorporate their pets in their family belief system (Beck & Katcher, 2003; Messent, 1983). The positive feelings we have toward nature in general and animals in particular are the human manifestation of our instincts as a social species living in the natural world (Beck & Katcher, 1996). There is an interesting consequence to our having positive feelings toward animals, as it also influences our feelings toward those associated with animals because of the fundamental attribution error. The fundamental attribution error (also correspondence bias) notes that there is a tendency for observers (us) to attribute other people's behavior to internal factors, such as liking animals, and to downplay situational causes, which are out of the observed person's control (Gilbert & Malone, 1995). People with animals are assumed to be better, more approachable people (Lockwood, 1983). People walking with their dog experience more social contact and longer conversations than when walking alone (McNicholas & Collis, 2000; Messent, 1983), and this may be especially important for people with visible disabilities who often encounter others who avoid eye contact, smiles, or conversation (Edelman, 1984; Kleck & Hastorf, 1966). Both child (Mader, Hart, & Bergin, 1989) and adult (Eddy, Hart, & Boltz, 1988) wheelchair users experienced significantly fewer of these avoidance behaviors if they were accompanied by a dog. Dog walkers will also experience the added joy of being approachable as they exercise.

This fascination with nature, especially pets, has developed into the study of the human-animal interaction (HAI), which is now an ever-expanding area of academic and clinical interest. From the beginning, the HAI concept had implications for improving both human and animal health. These studies, more than ever, have three distinct characteristics: (1) they are interdisciplinary, bringing together researchers from the disciplines of medicine, veterinary medicine, public health, nursing, psychology, social work, and education (Hines, 2003); (2) they are international in scope, with important centers of activity in the United Kingdom, France, Australia, Japan, Sweden, and North America; and (3) they are dispersed, that is, in addition to university researchers, there are many practitioners and independent scholars based outside the walls of academic environments such as veterinary practices, public health offices, high schools, prisons, therapeutic settings (like nursing homes), animal shelters, and volunteers. The people in the HAI field have always been dedicated to the translational nature of their work, that is, how the instincts, intuitions, and now research can be applied to human health (Beck, 2000; Friedmann & Thomas, 1995; Katcher & Beck, 2010).

Historically, the first organized application was the use of guide dogs for the blind (Ascarelli, 2010) and then non-service dogs brought to therapeutic settings, often with children with special needs or older adults in nursing homes (Beck & Katcher, 1984). Animal visitation to nursing homes and hospitals are becoming common, utilizing mostly dogs, though cats, llamas, small mammals, and even reptiles have had their place.

Recognizing the role of the pet dog for the non-institutionalized owner would appear obvious but only recently has the person-pet pair been an area of study (Beck & Katcher, 1996; Katcher, Friedmann, Beck, & Lynch, 1983; Siegel, 1990). In the presence of a dog people have been observed to be less stressed and have also been seen by others in a more positive way (Bauman, Russell, Furber, & Dobson, 2001; McNicholas & Collis, 2000; Rohlf, Toukhsati, Coleman, & Bennett, 2010; Thorpe et al., 2006a, 2006b).

Dog walking

Exercise has been one of the most useful tools to address one of society's most serious public health problem—obesity. There is a long history of programs and government guidelines addressing the obesity epidemic, from the 1970s programs focused mainly on diet, nutrition education, and encouraging physical activity. On this subject Nestle and Jacobson write, "Overall, the nearly half-century history of such banal recommendations is notable for addressing both physical activity and dietary patterns, but also for lack of creativity, a focus on individual behavior change, and ineffectiveness" (2000). There have been many programs but the obesity epidemic continues. We need to find an approach that people welcome, like harnessing animal lovers' natural commitment to their pets.

At first glance, dog walking does not seem a very difficult problem or cause for study. One only needs a dog that likes walking, which is almost every healthy dog, and an owner who also likes walking. Dog owners often walk more than those without dogs, and walking is one of the most basic ways to exercise. Dog walking is rapidly developing a whole new sub-discipline of the HAI community.

The real issue is convincing humans to want to walk with some regularity and creating the community infrastructure to make it easy and safe to take the walks. For that there has to be an honest assessment of the activity, so it warrants support and encouragement.

This book

Chapter 2 sets out the benefits of walking, presents national guidelines from several countries, looks at the United States in more detail, and finally discusses how dog walking may motivate walking as a physical activity. Chapters 3 and 8 review the evidence of the potential health benefits of dog walking, describe how dog walking could play a crucial role in improving human health, specifically through increasing amounts of daily physical activity, and explore how dog walking can be an enjoyable, economical, and effective weight management tool. Chapter 4 develops dog walking in the larger context of community integration, and chapter 5 focuses specifically on the value of walking for the older adult. Chapters 6, 7, and 10 present ways to encourage dog walking by discussing some actual programs. Chapter 11 describes research and practice directions needed to advance dog walking as a field.

We are now beginning to understand the relationship between dog ownership, physical activity, and human and animal health. Dog walking is a simple and enjoyable way to help dogs and ourselves.

References

Ascarelli, M. (2010). *Dorothy Harrison Eustis and the story of the Seeing Eye*. West Lafayette, IN: Purdue University Press.

Bauman, A. E., Russell, S. J., Furber, S. E., & Dobson, A. J. (2001). The epidemiology of dog walking: An unmet need for human and canine health. *Medical Journal of Australia, 175*(11-12), 632-634.

Beck, A. M. (2000). The use of animals to benefit humans, animal-assisted therapy. In A. H. Fine (Ed.), *The handbook on animal assisted therapy, theoretical foundations and guidelines for practice* (pp. 21-40). New York: Academic Press.

Beck, A. M., & Katcher, A. H. (1984). A new look at pet-facilitated therapy. *Journal of the American Veterinary Medicine Association, 184*, 414-421.

Beck, A. M., & Katcher, A. H. (1996). *Between pets and people: The importance of animal companionship*. West Lafayette, IN: Purdue University Press.

Beck, A. M., & Katcher, A. H. (2003). Future directions in human-animal bond research. *American Behavioral Scientist, 47*(1), 79-93.

Eddy, J., Hart, L. A, & Boltz, R. P. (1988). The effects of service dogs on social acknowledgements of people in wheelchairs. *The Journal of Psychology, 122*(1), 3945.

Edelman, R. J. (1984). Disablement and eye contact. *Perceptual and Motor Skills, 58*, 849-850.

Friedmann, E., & Thomas, S. A. (1995). Pet ownership, social support, and one-year survival after acute myocardial infarction in the cardiac arrhythmia suppression trial (CAST). *American Journal of Cardiology, 76*, 1213-1217.

Gilbert, D. T., & Malone, P. S. (1995). The correspondence bias. *Psychological Bulletin, 117*, 21-38.

Hawkley, L. C., & Cacioppo, J. T. (2007). Aging and loneliness: Downhill quickly? *Current Directions in Psychological Science, 16*, 187-191.

Hines, L. M. (2003). Historical perspective on the human-animal bond. *American Behavioral Scientist, 47*, 7-15.

Katcher, A. H., & Beck, A. M. (2010). The use of animals to benefit humans, animal-assisted therapy. In A. H. Fine (Ed.), *The handbook on animal-assisted therapy, and interventions* (pp. 49-58). New York: Academic Press.

Katcher, A. H., Friedmann, E., Beck, A. M., & Lynch, J. J. (1983). Looking, talking and blood pressure: The physiological consequences of interaction with the living environment. In A. H. Katcher & A. M. Beck (Eds.), *New perspectives on our lives with companion animals* (pp. 351-359). Philadelphia: University of Pennsylvania Press.

Kleck, R., Ono, H., & Hastorf, A. H. (1966). The effects of physical deviance on face-to-face interaction. *Human Relations, 19*(4), 425-436.

Lockwood, R. (1983). The influence of animals on social perception. In A. H. Katcher & A. M. Beck (Eds.), *New perspectives on our lives with companion animals* (pp. 64-71). Philadelphia: University of Pennsylvania Press.

Lynch, J. J. (1977). *The broken heart: The medical consequences of loneliness.* New York: Basic Books.

Lynch, J. J. (2000). *A cry unheard: New insights into the medical consequences of loneliness.* Baltimore, MD: Bancroft Press.

McNicholas, J., & Collis, G. M. (2000). Dogs as catalysts for social interactions: Robustness of the effect. *British Journal of Psychology, 91*, 61-70.

Mader, B., Hart, L. A., & Bergin, B. (1989). Social acknowledgments for children with disabilities: Effects of service dogs. *Child Development, 60*, 1529-1534.

Messent, P. R. (1983). Social facilitation of contact with other people by pet dogs. In A. H. Katcher & A. M. Beck (Eds.), *New perspectives on our lives with companion animals* (pp. 37-46). Philadelphia: University of Pennsylvania Press.

Nestle, M., & Jacobson, M. F. (2000). Halting the obesity epidemic: A public health policy approach. *Public Health Reports, 115*(1), 12-24.

Siegel, J. M. (1990). Stressful life events and use of physician services among the elderly: The moderating role of pet ownership. *Journal of Personality and Social Psychology, 58*, 1081-1086.

Thorpe, R. J., Kreisle, R. A, Glickman, L. T., Simonsick, E. M., Newman, A. B., & Kritchevsky, S. (2006a). Physical activity and pet ownership in year 3 of the Health ABC Study. *Journal of Aging and Physical Activity, 14*, 154-168.

Thorpe, R. J., Simonsick, E. M., Brach, J. S., Ayonayon, H., Satterfield, S., Harris, T. B., Garcia, M., & Kritchevsky, S. B. (2006b). Dog ownership, walking behavior, and maintained mobility in late life. *Journal American Geriatric Society, 54*, 1419-1424.

Rohlf, V. I., Toukhsati, S., Coleman, G. J., & Bennett, P. C. (2010). Dog obesity: Can dog caregivers' (owners') feeding and exercise intentions and behaviors be predicted from attitudes? *Journal of Animal Welfare Science, 13*, 213-236.

Weinick, R. M. (1998). Health-related behaviors and the benefits of marriage for elderly persons. *The Gerontologist, 38*, 618-627.

Wilson, E. O. (1993). Biophilia and the conservation ethic. In S. R. Kellert & E. O. Wilson (Eds.), *The biophilia hypothesis* (pp. 31-41). Washington, DC: Island Press.

Chapter 2

Physical activity recommendations and dog walking

Jacqueline N. Epping

Health benefits of physical activity: Why should we be active?

The health benefits of physical activity are numerous, significant, and well documented. People who are regularly physically active have better health and a lower risk of developing a variety of chronic diseases than people who are inactive. More active adults have lower rates of all-cause mortality, coronary artery disease, high blood pressure, stroke, type 2 diabetes, metabolic syndrome, colon cancer, breast cancer, and depression. Additionally, compared with less active people, physically active adults have higher levels of cardiorespiratory (aerobic) and muscular fitness, more favorable body composition and body mass, better quality sleep, and better health-related quality of life for older adults; regular physical activity is also associated with higher levels of functional health, lower risk of falls, and improved cognitive function. In children and youth, regular participation in physical activity is associated with better cardiorespiratory and muscular fitness, bone health, and body mass and composition (Physical Activity Guidelines Advisory Committee Report, 2008).

People who are the least active have the highest risk for a number of negative health outcomes, and evidence suggests that as little as one hour per week of moderate-to-vigorous physical activity can reduce risk of all-cause mortality and coronary artery disease (Physical Activity Guidelines Advisory Committee Report, 2008).

This chapter sets out the benefits of walking, presents national physical activity guidelines and recommendations from several countries, discusses physical activity prevalence, costs associated with inactivity, cost savings of regular physical activity, the relevance of dog walking in these contexts, and how dog walking may motivate walking as a physical activity.

The benefits of walking: Why is promoting walking a good strategy?

Although health and other benefits can be achieved by a variety of physical activities, the *2008 Physical Activity Guidelines for Americans* (http://www.health.gov/paguidelines/) notes specifically that a number of health and fitness benefits are derived from regular brisk walking, particularly for people who have been sedentary or physically active on an infrequent basis. An additional benefit of walking is that it is accessible to a large proportion of the population. This includes people for whom physical activities that have a cost, such as gym membership or organized sports, may be prohibitive. Walking is also accessible to people for whom physical access to facilities, programs, or equipment is limited or nonexistent. Walking is accessible to people of all ages, fitness levels, and abilities and requires no special equipment, program, or facility. It is a physical activity that can generally be performed safely even by previously sedentary individuals (Hootman et al., 2001).

Walking has been cited as the most common and popular form of physical activity among adults in the U.S. (Centers for Disease Control and Prevention, 1991), and in Canada, walking has been ranked as the most popular form of physical activity by 71% of the population of adults, age 20 and older (Statistics Canada, 2005).

Physical activity terminology: What does "active" mean?

National guidelines and recommendations for physical activity exist in a number of countries. In order to understand and effectively translate guidelines into behavior, it is important to understand some of the terminology typically used and associated with physical activity. For example, many guidelines and recommendations advocate moderate-to-vigorous physical activity, which refers to the intensity of the activity. The absolute intensity of physical activity is often described in terms of metabolic equivalents or METs. One MET is the rate of energy that one expends while sitting at rest. This is considered to be an oxygen uptake of 3.5 milliliters per kilogram of body weight per minute. Light-intensity activities are defined as 1.1 MET to 2.9 METs. Moderate-intensity activities are defined as 3.0 to 5.9 METs. Walking at 3 miles per hour ("a brisk walk") requires 3.3 METs of energy, thus is considered a moderate-intensity activity. Vigorous-intensity activities are defined as 6.0 METs or more. For example, running at 6 miles per hour (10 minutes per mile) requires10 METs of energy expenditure, so running at that rate is considered as vigorous-intensity (*2008 Physical Activity Guidelines for Americans*). Intensity can also be described in relative terms. A simple way to gauge relative intensity is by the level of effort required. Less fit people typically require a higher level of effort than people who are fitter to do the same activity. A scale of 0 to 10 can be used to estimate relative intensity, where 0 is equivalent to sitting and 10 is the highest level of effort possible. Moderate-intensity activity is at a level of 5 or 6; vigorous-intensity activity is at a level of 7 or 8. Using relative intensity, during moderate-intensity activity a person can talk but not sing. A person doing vigorous-intensity activity can only say a few words without needing to take a breath (*2008 Physical Activity Guidelines for Americans*). Similarly, moderate-intensity activity would not cause most people to "break a sweat," but vigorous-intensity activity would cause sweating.

Physical activity guidelines and recommendations: How active should we be?

In the United Kingdom, the recommendation for adults is 30 minutes per day on five or more days of the week, and for children it is 60 minutes per day on five or more days of the week (Department of Health, 2004). The government has set targets in England and Wales for 70% of the population to be "reasonably active" by 2020. The target in Scotland is for 50% of adults to achieve the minimum levels by 2022 (Department of Health, 2004; Welsh Assembly Government, 2003).

The National Physical Activity Guidelines for adults in Australia recommend at least 30 minutes of moderate-intensity activity (including brisk walking) on most days of the week, with each session lasting at least 10 minutes. This is generally interpreted as 30 minutes at least five days of the week, a total of 150 minutes of moderate-intensity activity per week. Children are recommended to do 60 minutes of moderate-to-vigorous physical activity every day *(*Australian Institute of Health and Welfare, 2006)

In Japan, the recommendation is approximately 60 minutes of physical activity at an intensity of 3.3 METs, that is, 3.3 times the intensity of being at rest (e.g., sitting). This is at an intensity equivalent to walking for most people. This level of physical activity is recommended to be performed seven days per week for a total of 420 minutes per week (Shibata, Koichiro, Harada, Nakamura, & Muraoka, 2009).

Physical activity guidelines for North Americans: What is our aim?

In the U.S., Healthy People Objectives are 10-year national objectives for promoting health and preventing disease. Every decade, the U.S. Department of Health and Human Services (HHS) establishes new objectives that are developed through a broad consultation process, including public comment. They are built on the best scientific knowledge and knowledge of current data, trends, and innovations, and are designed to measure programs over time. *Healthy People 2020* (http://www.healthypeople.gov/hp2020/) includes 14 objectives for physical activity and fitness (Table 2.1):

Table 2.1. Healthy People 2020 Objectives.

1. Reduce the proportion of adults who engage in no leisure-time physical activity.

2. Increase the proportion of the Nation's public and private schools that require daily physical education for all students.

3. Increase the proportion of adolescents who participate in daily school physical education.

4. Increase the proportion of adolescents who spend at least 50 percent of school physical education class time being physically active.

5. Increase the proportion of the Nation's public and private schools that provide access to their physical activity spaces and facilities for all persons outside of normal school hours.

6. Increase the proportion of adults that meet current Federal physical activity guidelines for aerobic physical activity and for muscle strength training.

7. Increase the proportion of adolescents that meet current physical activity guidelines for aerobic physical activity and for muscle-strengthening activity.

8. Increase the proportion of children and adolescents that meet guidelines for television viewing and computer use.

9. Increase the proportion of employed adults who have access to and participate in employer-based exercise facilities and exercise programs.

10. Increase the proportion of trips made by walking.

11. Increase the proportion of trips made by bicycling.

12. Increase the proportion of States and school districts that require regularly scheduled elementary school recess.

13. Increase the proportion of school districts that require or recommend elementary school recess for an appropriate period of time.

14. Increase the proportion of physician office visits for chronic health diseases or conditions that include counseling or education related to exercise.

Dog walking has potential for helping meet four Healthy People Objectives in particular: Objective 1, decreasing the number of adults reporting no leisure-time physical activity; Objective 6 and Objective 7, increasing the proportion of adults and adolescents who meet physical activity guidelines; and Objective 10, increasing walking trips.

The first guidelines for physical activity in the U.S. were published in 1972 by the American Heart Association. Since that time a number of guidelines and Position Stands have been published, including Position Stands issued by the American College of Sports Medicine (ACSM) in 1978, 1990, and 1998. Earlier physical activity guidelines focused on the clinical assessment of exercise capacity or on the development of cardiorespiratory (aerobic) fitness and body composition, that is, the recommendations were designed to achieve, increase, or maintain levels of physical fitness, and generally recommended vigorous-intensity physical activity. For example, the 1978 ACSM Position Stand on "The Recommended Quantity and Quality of Exercise for Developing and Maintaining Fitness in Healthy Adults" recommended 15 to 60 minutes of an endurance-type activity, 3 to 5 days per week, at a level of 60% to 90% of heart rate reserve or 50% to 85% of maximal oxygen uptake.

A major shift in focus from fitness-related physical activity recommendations to health-related physical activity recommendations occurred with the 1995 release of *Physical Activity and Public Health: A Recommendation from the Centers for Disease Control and Prevention and the American College of Sports Medicine*. The primary recommendation of this report was that all adults should accumulate 30 minutes or more of moderate-intensity physical activity (an intensity 3.0 to 5.9 times the intensity of rest) on most, preferably all, days of the week (Pate et al., 1995). This represented a significant change from earlier guidelines, not only in terms of the levels of physical activity recommended, but also in shifting focus from guidelines that only a relatively small proportion of the population was meeting to guidelines that more of the population might be able to aspire to and meet (Physical Activity Guidelines Advisory Committee, 2008). Shortly after the CDC/ACSM report, the National Institutes of Health (NIH) and World Health Organization (WHO) issued reports on the health benefits of regular physical activity, and in 1996 *Physical Activity and Health: A Report of the Surgeon General* was issued, which recommended that people of all ages could improve health and quality of life by participating in lifelong moderate-intensity physical activity (U.S. Department of Health and Human Services, 1996). Since that time, the body of knowledge of the wide range of health benefits from participation in physical activity has grown substantially, and in 2008 the first comprehensive federal guidelines on physical activity, the *2008 Physical Activity Guidelines for Americans*, were issued. Key guidelines are included for children and adolescents, adults, older adults, women during pregnancy and the postpartum period, and adults with disabilities. Key messages for people with chronic medical conditions, guidelines for safe physical activity, and recommendations for how various levels of society can support individuals in being physically active are also included.

A key recommendation for both adults and older adults is to avoid inactivity, including prolonged sitting. Even bouts of 10 minutes of moderate-to-vigorous physical activity provides health benefits (Dunn et al., 1998), and even light activity (defined as less than 3 METs) contributes significantly to energy expenditure (Owen, Healy, Matthews, & Dunstan, 2010). In simple terms, this could translate into taking three 10 minute walks a day, for example, one in the morning, one at lunchtime, and one at the end of the work day or in the evening. In terms of health benefits, an important and fundamental message is that some activity is better than none, and more is better. The most important measure of how much physical activity to perform is the total volume of physical activity per week. This, unlike earlier guidelines that specified physical activity intensity, duration, and frequency, allows individuals the flexibility to meet the guidelines a number of different ways.

In addition to guidelines for individuals, a chapter is included with recommendations for how individuals can be supported in being physically active by various societal levels and sectors. In addition to addressing physical activity at the individual level, it is also addressed at various levels of behavioral influence, including families and communities. For example, communities are encouraged to provide opportunities for physical activity and to use evidence-based intervention strategies, including those recommended by the U.S. Task Force on Community Preventive Services in 2002. Some of strategies are particularly relevant to, and provide rationale for, dog walking as a potentially effective intervention strategy. They are discussed later in this chapter.

The U.S. national physical activity plan: How are we going to get where we want to go in the U.S.?

The first National Physical Activity Plan (NPAP) was launched May 3, 2010.

The plan was established in recognition of the need for a broad, comprehensive framework from which to promote physical activity. Development of the plan was informed by other physical activity plans around the world, including plans from Western Australia, Canada, Finland, Northern Ireland, Pakistan and the United Kingdom (www.physicalactivityplan.org/NationalPhysical ActivityPlan.pdf).

A primary mission of the plan is to produce a marked and progressive increase in the percentage of Americans who meet physical activity guidelines throughout life. The goals of the plan are to:

1. "Make a compelling and urgent case for increasing physical activity in the American population;

2. Provide a clear roadmap for actions that support short and long-term progress in increasing Americans' physical activity;

3. Develop strategies for increasing physical activity in all population subgroups and reducing disparities across subgroups;

4. Create a sustained and resourced social movement that provides for ongoing coordination, partnerships, capacity building, and evaluation;

5. Develop new and innovative strategies for promoting physical activity;

6. Undergo periodic evaluation to assess achievements in increasing physical activity."

The goal to develop new and innovative strategies for promoting physical activity (point 5 in the plan) is directly relevant to dog walking as a promoter of physical activity. Promoting and facilitating dog walking is a new and innovative strategy that could help Americans meet physical activity guidelines throughout life, and dog walking has shown promise in increasing physical activity and improving various dimensions of health in subgroups of the general population, including older adults (Thorpe et al., 2006), disadvantaged individuals (Johnson & Meadows, 2010), and youth (Wright and Brown, 2011).

Prevalence of physical activity: How active are we?

Despite the health benefits of regular physical activity, including the benefits of walking, and the potential negative health outcome of physical inactivity, at least 60% of the global population does not achieve recommended levels of physical activity. The global estimate for the prevalence of physical inactivity among adults is 17%. Estimates for prevalence of some, but insufficient, activity (less than 2.5 hours per week of moderate activity) range from 31% to 51%, with a global average of 41% (WHO, http://www.who.int/dietphysicalactivity/en/).

In the United Kingdom, only 40% of men and 28% of women meet the minimum recommendations for adults (NHS Information Centre, 2008). From 1997 to 2006, 30% to 35% of adults in the United States reported being physically active at moderate- or vigorous-intensity sufficient to meet existing recommendations. Thirty-five to forty percent reported no leisure time physical activity (CDC 2010, available from http://wonder.cdc.gov/data2010). Less than 20% of U.S. students in grades 9 through 12 reported meeting moderate-to-vigorous intensity physical activity recommendations, according to data from the 2009 Youth Risk Behavior Surveillance System (YRBSS, 2009).

What is the cost of being inactive?

The health problems associated with physical inactivity are the leading causes of death in developed countries (WHO, 2002). Globally inactivity has been estimated to cause 1.9 million deaths per year (Cobiac, Vos, & Barendregt, 2009). It is estimated to cause about 10% to 16% of cases of breast cancer, colon cancer, and diabetes, and about 22% of ischemic heart disease (WHO, http://www.who.int/dietphysicalactivity/en/). In Australia, physical inactivity leads to 10% of all deaths, largely as a result of cardiovascular disease and diabetes. Time viewing television, in particular, has been inversely associated with undiagnosed abnormal glucose metabolism and the metabolic syndrome, independent of waist circumference (Owen, Healy, Matthews, & Dunstan, 2010). In the U.S., unhealthy lifestyle, which includes physical inactivity, is the primary contributor to the six leading causes of death—heart disease, cancer, stroke, respiratory diseases, accidents, and diabetes—which collectively account for over 70% of all deaths (Anderson & Smith, 2005). The prevalence of obesity among U.S. adults rose to 30% in 1999-2000, a 33% increase from a decade earlier (Flegal, Carroll, Ogden, & Johnson, 2002), and the prevalence of diabetes also rose by 33% during approximately the same period (Mokdad et al., 2000). About one-third of American adults are obese (Flegal, Carroll, Ogden & Curtin, 2010).

In addition to the human cost of suffering in terms of illness, disability, and death, physical inactivity results in tremendous economic costs. For example, the cost of physical inactivity in England, including direct medical cost treatment for related diseases and the indirect cost caused through absences due to sickness, has been estimated at £8.2 billion per year, not including the contribution of inactivity to the cost of obesity, which itself is estimated to be £2.5 billion per year (Department of Health, 2004). The Australian Bureau of Statistics estimated annual direct health care costs attributable to physical inactivity to be around $377AUS million per year (2006). The overall annual direct medical costs of inactivity (in 2000 dollars) in the U.S. have been estimated to be $76.6 billion (Pratt, Macera, & Wang, 2000). In Canada, physical inactivity accounts for about 6% of total health care costs (WHO, http://www.who.int/dietphysicalactivity/publications/facts/pa/en/).

What are the cost savings of physical activity?

A review of the medical expenditures of over 35,000 U.S. adults revealed that medical expenditures for physically active adults were approximately $1,000 less annually than those for inactive adults, and estimated a cost savings of $76.6 billion (in 2000 dollars) if all inactive Americans became physically active (Pratt, Macera, & Wang, 2000) A 25% reduction in death from coronary artery disease has been estimated as a result of the impact of physical activity as a lifestyle change, which is comparable to drug therapies (Iestra et al., 2005). An annual cost savings of approximately $5 billion could be realized if 10% of the sedentary population in the U.S. would adopt a walking program (Jones & Easton, 1994). Findings from an epidemiological study of dog walking in Australia estimated that if all dog owners walked their dogs more, the result would be a 24% increase nationally in adults who are considered to be sufficiently active, and a direct health care cost savings of around $175AUS million per year (Bauman, Russell, Furber, & Dobson, 2001).

Determinants and correlates of physical activity: What moves us to move?

Understanding what motivates people to be active is an important prerequisite for designing relevant and effective programs (Shibata, Koichiro, Harada, Nakamura, & Muraoka, 2009). Psychological (intrapersonal), social (interpersonal), and environmental factors all influence physical activity behavior. Intrapersonal factors include knowledge, attitudes, beliefs, motivation, self-concept, developmental history, past experience, and skills. Interpersonal factors include the opinions, thoughts, behavior, advice, and support of those surrounding an individual (*Theory at a Glance: A Guide for Health Promotion Practice*, 2005). The ecological perspective of health behavior change emphasizes the interaction between, and interdependence of, factors within and across all levels of influence. This perspective posits that individual behavior both shapes and is shaped by the social environment (Smedley & Syme, 2000).

Shibata and Koichiro (2009) found that self-efficacy (one's belief in one's ability to perform an activity or engage in a behavior), possessing home fitness equipment, having social support, and having access to enjoyable scenery were all positively associated with achieving recommended levels of physical activity. In a review of 24 studies that examined variables influencing physical activity, physical activity self-efficacy was the most consistent intrapersonal correlate of physical activity behavior. Social support was also a consistently important interpersonal correlate. Physical environment correlates that were positively associated with physical activity included having exercise equipment at home or having access to facilities (Trost, Owen, Bauman, & Sallis, 2002). Lian et al. found that, among older adults, lack of an exercise partner and no access to facilities were among the most significant barriers to physical activity (1999). These findings have implications for why dog walking may be effective in promoting physical activity. Dogs can be regular and loyal exercise partners and provide social support that can increase self-efficacy for being physically active. Additionally, dogs could be viewed as "exercise equipment" that are readily available, thus providing easy access to opportunities for physical activity. Finally, community-based programs such as the Walk a Hound, Lose a Pound programs in Lubbock, Texas, Columbia, Missouri (Johnson & McKenney, 2010, *http://rechai.missouri.edu/rp.htm)*, and Indianapolis, Indiana (www.walkahound.org/) create access to additional opportunities for physical activity, including opportunities for people without dogs. These programs provide community volunteers the opportunity to walk homeless dogs, including dogs that are in shelters. Many people may not be able to have their own dogs for a variety of reasons. For example, housing facilities such as college dorms or apartments may not allow dogs. Resources to care full-time for a dog, including the necessary time, may be a barrier for some people. Programs such as Walk a Hound, Lose a Pound provide an opportunity for these people to be physically active, share the companionship of a dog, and volunteer in their communities.

Public health physical activity intervention recommendations: What population-based intervention approaches can get us moving?

Given the public health importance of increasing physical activity at the population level, effective, feasible intervention approaches and strategies to increase physical activity are needed. They need to be applicable to large segments of the population and be sustainable in community settings. The U.S. Task Force on Community Preventive Services has recommended several such intervention approaches, based on systematic reviews of the scientific evidence of effectiveness, published in *The Guide to Community Preventive Services* (Zaza, Briss, & Harris, 2005) Because increasing physical activity involves behavioral, social, and environmental factors (both physical and social environments), the recommended approaches are grouped into three general domains: informational approaches, behavioral and social approaches, and environmental and policy approaches.

Within the domain of informational approaches, two interventions are recommended: community-wide campaigns and point-of-decision prompts (signs at elevators and escalators that encourage stair use). Recommended interventions within the behavioral and social approaches include school-based physical education, individually-adapted health behavior change programs, and social support interventions in community settings. Interventions recommended within environmental and policy approaches include creation of or enhanced access to places for physical activity combined with informational outreach activities, community-scale urban design and land use policies and practices, and street-scale urban design and land use policies and practices.

Of these recommendations, three may have particular relevance to dog walking as an approach to increase physical activity: individually adapted health behavior change programs, social support in community settings, and creation of or enhanced access to places for physical activity combined with informational outreach activities.

Individually adapted health behavior change programs are tailored to individuals' specific interests, preferences, and readiness to change, and involve behavioral skills that allow individuals to make moderate-intensity physical activity part of their daily routines. Skills may include recognizing cues and opportunities for physical activity and building social support for becoming physically active, among others. Dogs can provide both cues and opportunities for being physically active as part of a daily or regular routine, dog walking can support moderate-intensity physical activity, and dogs may provide social support that can help reinforce the adoption and maintenance of regular physical activity.

Interventions that employ social support in community settings build, strengthen, and maintain social networks that support increased physical activity. These interventions typically create buddy systems, which make contracts among the buddies to create expectations and accountability, and/or form groups, such as walking groups, to provide companionship and support while being physically active. Dogs can create expectations and accountability for regular physical activity (think of your dog waiting at the door to go for a walk). They can also provide companionship, enjoyment, a sense of increased safety, and social support. In these ways, dogs may be able to increase individual's motivation and self-efficacy for being physically active.

The creation of or enhanced access to places for physical activity combined with informational outreach activities may have a relationship to dog walking both in terms of encouraging dog owners to walk—or walk more—with their dogs, and in terms of community volunteer dog walking programs such as the Walk a Hound, Lose a Pound programs. Although this particular intervention approach was identified and recommended from the findings of studies that created or increased access to *places* for physical activity, it is reasonable to assert that a fundamental element of this strategy is to create or increase access to *opportunities* for physical activity, whether or not those opportunities are reflected in physical structures. Having, or having access to, a dog could be considered creating or enhancing access to physical activity opportunities by virtue of the dog; that is, dog walking creates an opportunity for activity that would not exist without the dog. From this perspective, encouraging dog owners to walk more with their dogs enhances their opportunities to be physically active. In the case of community-based volunteer dog walking program—such as Walk a Hound, Lose a Pound—access to both places and opportunities for physical activity are provided via the program and facilities in which it is conducted, and may reach both dog owners and non-dog owners.

Encouraging dog owners who do walk their dogs to walk more holds great promise for increasing physical activity at the population level, given that a significant proportion of households in many developed countries include dogs. For example, nearly 40% of U.S. households include at least one dog (Ham & Epping, 2006). This is similar to the rates in Australia (Bauman et al., 2001). Nearly 38% of households in France include at least one dog (*Dog Business Digest*, October, 2002). However, not all dog owners walk their dogs. For example, an Australian study (Bauman et al., 2001) found that over half of dog owners did not walk their dogs, and these owners were actually less likely than non-dog owners to meet recommended levels of physical activity, so encouraging dog owners who do not walk their dogs should also be considered an important strategy to increase physical activity on a large scale.

Purposeful physical activity: How might we sustain healthy levels of physical activity?

William P. Morgan (2001) noted that adherence to formal exercise programs has averaged around 50% over the past decades, and he attributed this to the "non-purposeful" approaches that characterize many formal exercise programs. He called for a paradigm shift in the prescription of physical activity to one characterized by "purposeful" activity. Ten case studies of individuals ranging in age from 35 years to 85 years were examined and described. These individuals reported participation in "purposeful" physical activity from between 5 years and 79 years, and walking between 3 to 8 miles per day, with a minimum of five days per week in each case. Three of the case studies were of dog walkers. One 60-year-old dog walker reported walking 3 miles per day for approximately 10 years; one 55-year-old dog walker reported walking 4 miles per day for approximately 15 years; and one 35-year-old dog walker reported walking 6 miles per day for approximately 5 years. The physical activity levels of these dog walkers exceed current U.S. physical activity guidelines. The dog walkers reported that they walked on a daily basis primarily because their dogs needed the exercise (Morgan, 2001). The amount of physical activity reported by the dog walkers in this study indicates that dogs can be powerful motivators of physical activity in terms of a sense of obligation to provide the dogs with exercise.

The association of dog walking and meeting physical activity guidelines: What does the research say?

The epidemiology of dog walking for fitness and health is addressed in detail in chapter 3; however, it is worth noting that epidemiological studies suggest that dog walking may not only help individuals increase and sustain regular physical activity, but may help people meet and sustain *recommended* levels of physical activity. For example, Thorpe et al. (2006) found that, among older adults, dog walkers were more likely to meet physical activity recommendations of 150 minutes per week through walking than dog owners who did not walk their dogs. Three years later, the dog walkers were twice as likely to achieve that same level of physical activity as either dog owners who did not walk their dogs or non-dog owners. Additionally, the dog walkers had faster usual and rapid walking speeds than dog owners who did not walk their dogs (Thorpe et al., 2006). An analysis of data from the National Household Travel Survey in the United States showed that, in one day, nearly 43% of dog walkers accumulated at least 30 minutes of physical activity from walks lasting at least 10 minutes each (Ham & Epping, 2006). Unpublished data from the U.S. HealthStyles survey showed that dog owners were approximately 30% more likely to meet physical activity recommendations of 150 minutes per week than non-dog owners (Epping & Yore).

Conclusion

Physical activity guidelines have been developed in a number of countries, based on reviews of the scientific evidence. Effective population-based intervention strategies to promote physical activity are important to support individuals in meeting these guidelines. Developing and implementing practical and sustainable strategies with sufficient reach to shift participation in health-enhancing physical activities at the population level is challenging. While the evidence for dog walking has not yet been sufficient to include as a recommended strategy, the research in this area is growing. As the research grows and, in particular, as additional evidence from intervention studies emerges, dog walking may well be among specific strategies that are recommended and that can help a large proportion of the population meet physical activity guidelines and recommendations.

References

American Heart Association. Committee on Exercise. Exercise testing and training of apparently healthy individuals: A handbook for physicians. (1972). Dallas, TX: American Heart Association.

American College of Sports Medicine position statement on the recommended quantity and quality of exercise for developing and maintaining fitness in healthy adults. (1978). *Medicine & Science in Sports & Exercise, 10*(3), vii-vix.

American College of Sports Medicine position statement on the recommended quantity and quality of exercise for developing and maintaining fitness in healthy adults. (1990). *Medicine & Science in Sports & Exercise, 22*(2), 265-274.

American College of Sports Medicine position statement on the recommended quantity and quality of exercise for developing and maintaining fitness in healthy adults. (1998). *Medicine & Science in Sports & Exercise, 30*(6), 975-991.

Anderson, R. N, & Smith, B. L. (2005). Deaths: Leading causes for 2002. National Vital Statistics Report. *National Center for Health Statistics, 53*(17).

Australian Institute of Health and Welfare. (2006). Australia's health 2006. AIHW cat. no. AUS 73. Canberra: AIHW.

Australian Bureau of Statistics. (2006). 4835.0.55.001—Physical activity in Australia: A snapshot, 2004-05.

Bauman, A. E., Russell, S. J., Furber, S. E., & Dobson, A. J. (2001). The epidemiology of dog walking: An unmet need for human and canine health. *Medical Journal of Australia, 175*(11-12), 632-634.

Centers for Disease Control and Prevention. Prevalence of physical activity, including lifestyle activities among adults—United States, 2000-2001. (2003). *MMWR, 52*(32), 764-769.

Centers for Disease Control and Prevention. National Center for Health Statistics. (1991). National health interview statistics. Retrieved from http://www.cdc.gov/nchs/nhis.htm

Centers for Disease Control and Prevention. Data 2010: The Healthy People 2010 Database. (2008). Retrieved from http://wonder.cdc.gov/data2010

Cobiac, L. J., Vos, T., & Barendregt, J. J. (2009). Cost-effectiveness of interventions to promote physical activity: A modeling study. *PLoS Med 6*(7). e1000110. DOI:10.1371/journal.pmed.1000110.

Department of Health. (2004). At least five a week—Evidence on the impact of physical activity and its relationship to health—a report from the Chief Medical Officer. Retrieved from http://www.dh.gov.uk/en/Publicationsandstatistics/Publications/PublicationsPolicyAndGuidance/DH_4080994

Dog Business Digest. The dog market. October 2002. Retrieved from http://www.dog-digest.com/html/oct2002.html#1

Dunn, A. L., Garcia, M. E., Marcus, B. H., Kampert, J.B., Kohl, H. W., III, & Blair, S. N. (1998). Six-month physical activity and fitness changes in Project Active, a randomized trial. *Medicine & Science in Sports & Exercise, 30*, 1076-1083.

Epping, J., & Yore, M., unpublished.

Flegal, K.M., Carroll, M.D., Ogden, C.L., & Curtain, L.R. (2010). Prevalence and trends in obesity among US adults, 1999-2008. *JAMA, 303*(3), 235-241.

Ham, S. A., & Epping, J. Dog walking and physical activity in the United States. *Preventing Chronic Disease* [serial online] 2006 April. Retrieved from http:www.cdc.gov/pcd/issues/2006/apr/05_0106.htm

Healthy People 2020. Retrieved from http://www.healthypeople.gov/hp2020/. Accessed 1/31/2011.

Hootman, J., Macera, C., Ainsworth, B., Martin, M., Addy, C., & Blair, S. (2001). Association among physical activity level, cardiorespiratory fitness, and risk of musculoskeletal injury. *American Journal of Epidemiology, 154*(3), 251-258.

Iestra, J. A., Kromhout, D., van der Schouw, Y. T., Grobbee, D. E., Boshuizen, H. C., & van Staveren, W. A. (2005). Effect size estimates of lifestyle and dietary changes on all-cause mortality in coronary artery disease patients: A systematic review. *Circulation, 112*, 924-934.

Johnson, R. A., & Meadows, R. L. (2010). Dog walking: Motivation for adherence to a walking program. *Clinical Nursing Research, 19*(4), 387-402.

Johnson, R. A., & McKenney, C. (2010). Implementing a community fitness program involving shelter dogs: Issues & outcomes. Paper presentation at 14ᵗʰ International Conference on Human-Animal Interactions, International Association of Human Animal Interaction Organizations, Stockholm, Sweden.

Jones, T., & Easton, C. (1994). Cost-benefit analysis of walking to prevent coronary heart disease. *Archives of Family Medicine, 3,* 703-710.

Lian, W., Gan, G., Pin, C., Wee, S. & Ye, C. (1999). Correlates of leisure-time physical activity in an elderly population in Singapore. *American Journal of Public Health, 89,* 1578-1580.

Mokdad, A. H., Ford, E. S., Bowman, B. A., Nelson, D. E., Engelgau, M. M., Vinicor, F., & Marks, J. S. (2000). Diabetes trends in the U.S.: 1990–1998. *Diabetes Care, 23,* 1278-1283.

Morgan, W. (2001). Prescription of physical activity: A paradigm shift. *QUEST, 53,* 366-382.

Health survey for England 2006: CVD and risk factors adults, obesity and risk factors children. (2008). NHS Information Centre. Retrieved from http://www.ic.nhs.uk/pubs/hse06cvdandriskfactors

Owen, N., Healy, G. N., Matthews, C. E., & Dunstan, D. W. (2010). Too much sitting: The population health science of sedentary behavior. *Exercise and Sport Sciences Reviews, 38*(3), 105-113.

Pate, R. R., Pratt, M., Blair, S. N., Haskell, W. L., Macera, C. A., Bouchard, C., Buchner, D., Ettinger, W., Heath, G.W. & King, A.C. (1995). Physical activity and public health: A recommendation from the Centers for Disease Control and Prevention and the American College of Sports Medicine. *Journal of the American Medical Association, 2273*(5), 402-407.

Physical Activity Guidelines for Americans. (2008). ODPHP Publication NoU0036. Retrieved from www.health.gov/paguidelines.

Physical Activity Guidelines Advisory Committee. (2008). Physical activity guidelines advisory committee report. Washington, DC: Department of Health and Human Services.

Pratt, M., Macera, C., & Wang, G. (2000). Higher direct medical costs associated with physical inactivity. *Physician and Sports Medicine, 28*(10), 63-70.

Shibata, A., Koichiro, O., Harada, K., Nakamura, Y., & Muraoka, I. (2009). Psychological, social and environmental factors to meeting physical activity recommendations among Japanese adults. *International Journal of Behavioral Nutrition and Physical Activity, 6*(60), 1-12.

Smedley, B., & Syme, S. (Eds.). (2000). Institute of Medicine. Promoting health: Strategies from social and behavioral research. Washington, DC: National Academies Press.

Statistics Canada's Canadian Community Health Survey, Cycle 3.1. (2005). Retrieved from http://www.viha.ca/mho/stats_and_maps/Canadian+Community+Health+Survey.htm

Task Force on Community Preventive Services. (2002). Recommendations to increase physical activity: A systematic review. *American Journal of Preventive Medicine, 22*(4S), 67-72.

Theory at a glance: A guide for health promotion practice, 2nd ed. (2005). U.S. Department of Health and Human Services. National Institutes of Health. National Cancer Institute.

Thorpe, R. J., Kreisle, R. A., Glickman, L. T., Simonsick, E. M., Newman, A. B., & Kritchevsky, S. (2006). Physical activity and pet ownership in year 3 of the Health ABC Study. *Journal of Aging and Physical Activity, 14*, 154-168.

Thorpe, R., Simonsick, E. M., Brach, J. S., Ayonayon, H., Satterfield, S., Tamara B. Harris, T. B., Kritchevsky, S. B. (2006). Dog ownership, walking behavior, and maintained mobility in late life. *Journal of American Geriatric Society, 54*, 1419–1424.

Trost, S., Owen, N., Bauman, A. E., & Sallis, J. F. (2002). Correlates of adults' participation in physical activity: Review and update. *Medicine & Science in Sports & Exercise, 34*(12), 1996-2001.

U. S. Department of Agriculture (2009). Japan market development reports: Pet food 2009. Retrieved January 31, 2011, from http://www.fas.usda.gov/gainfiles/200905/146347788.pdf

U.S. Department of Health and Human Services. (1996). Physical activity and health: A report of the Surgeon General. Atlanta, GA: Dept. of Health and Human Services, Centers for Disease Control and Prevention, National Center for Chronic Disease Prevention and Health Promotion.

Welsh Assembly Government. (2003). Climbing higher—Strategy for sport and active recreation in Wales. Retrieved from http://wales.gov.uk/topics/cultureandsport/sportandactiverecreation/climbing/?lang=en

World Health Organization. Global strategy on diet, physical activity and health. Retrieved from http://www.who.int/dietphysicalactivity/strategy/eb11344/strategy_english_web.pdf

World Health Organization. (2002). The World Health report 2002—Reducing risks, promoting healthy life. Retrieved from http://www.who.int/whr/2002/en/whr02_en.pdf

Wright, K. K., & Brown, A. M. (2011, in press). Kids and K-9s for healthy choices: A pilot program for canine therapy and healthy behavior modification to increase healthy lifestyle choices in children. In R. A. Johnson, A. M. Beck, & S. McCune. *The health benefits of dog walking* (ch. 10). West Lafayette, IN: Purdue University Press.

Youth Risk Behavior Surveillance System. (2009). 2009 national Youth Risk Behavior Survey Overview. Retrieved from http://www.cdc.gov/HealthyYouth

Zaza, S., Briss, P., & Harris, K. W. (Eds.). (2005). The guide to community preventive services: What works to promote health? New York: Oxford University Press.

Chapter 3

International perspectives on the epidemiology of dog walking

Adrian Bauman, Hayley E. Christian, Roland J. Thorpe, Jr., and Rona Macniven

Physical activity promotes and improves human health. Despite this, many populations remain physically inactive, with limited or no changes in activity patterns over recent decades. One possible solution is to encourage dog walking, with high rates of dog ownership in many countries. This chapter describes the potential for dog walking to improve human health, through improvements in physical activity.

The health benefits of physical activity

Regular moderate-intensity physical activity is an important contributor to overall population health. In particular, the best available epidemiological evidence suggests that accumulating at least 30 minutes each day of moderate-intensity physical activity can contribute to a range of health benefits, particularly preventing many chronic diseases. This quantum of physical activity has a strong protective effect in reducing the risk of cardiovascular disease and type 2 diabetes (USDHHS, 2008). In addition, physical activity favorably impacts upon health in the elderly, improves cognition, reduces the risk of dementia, and reduces the risk of falls among older adults (Nelson et al., 2007). For all people, physical activity has mental health and social benefits, improving quality of life, preventing anxiety, depression, and reducing stress levels (Haskell et al., 2007; USDHHS, 2008). The social benefits include increasing community engagement, creating community social capital, fostering social interaction, and contributing to a healthier social and physical environment (Wood, Giles-Corti, & Bulsara, 2005).

Overall, physical inactivity ranks equally with tobacco smoking, high blood pressure, high cholesterol, or obesity as a threat to population health, particularly in developed and transitional countries (WHO, 2009). Despite this evidence, physical activity receives less attention from the media, from decision makers, and from health professionals than the other major risk factors (Chau, Bonfiglioli, Chey, & Bauman, 2009). Thus, it is particularly important to establish and develop effective approaches to increase population-levels of regular physical activity.

Distillation of the epidemiological evidence suggests that adults need "at least 30 minutes of moderate intensity physical activity per day" (USDHHS, 2008). More activity than this will confer slightly additional health benefits, and strength training is important for the elderly, but the greatest population benefit will occur when completely sedentary or very inactive individuals increase their activity levels to reach the "30 minutes per day" threshold. This threshold is embodied in recent global physical activity guidelines and recommendations (WHO, 2010).

An important dimension to consider is the health implications of total daily energy expenditure. Human beings are healthier if they "move more" and spend less time sitting. This is important with respect to obesity prevention, as the total energy expended throughout the day will act to counterbalance increases in energy (food) intake (Bauman, Allman-Farinelli, Huxley, & James, 2008). The public health recommendation for obesity prevention requires more physical activity than the minimal recommendation of 30 minutes per day. Typically 60-90 minutes of physical activity per day is suggested for weight maintenance or weight loss. For this reason, multiple settings for increasing physical activity, most likely through walking, can add to daily energy expenditure in useful ways to prevent obesity.

The challenge of public health practitioners is to increase physical activity across large segments of the population, not just those that can afford to access gyms, structured programs, and personal trainers. While there is ample evidence that structured exercise programs are effective in increasing activity among those that participate, there has been less success in achieving whole population changes in physical activity. For this reason, the public health challenge remains to develop physical activity strategies that transcend age, gender, and cultural groups, and that are accessible and affordable to all within the population. For example, walking has been shown to be the most popular form of physical activity; behaviorally, it is easy, requires little financial outlay, and can be done almost anywhere and at any time by anybody (Bauman, Bellew, Vita, Brown, & Owen, 2002).

In this context, dog walking has substantial public health potential, because of the reach, accessibility, and type of moderate-intensity physical activity involved. This chapter describes the evidence base for the assertion that human health could be improved substantially if all of those who owned dogs increased the amount of walking they did with their dog.

The public health potential for dog walking

A public health approach first describes the magnitude of the problem, and then identifies potential solutions, and the benefits that might arise if prevention programs were fully implemented. The first task here is to describe rates of meeting "physical activity recommendations" across different countries. This is the proportion of the (adult) population that meets the 30 minutes per day of physical activity recommended to achieve the defined health benefits. The arguments for dog walking to increase physical activity here are confined to adults, and the more complex area of adolescent and children's physical activity, or their role in walking with their dog, is not addressed here, but is an emerging area of research (Owen et al., 2010; Timperio, Salmon, Chu, & Veitch, 2008).

A review of physical activity prevalence studies is shown in Table 3.1. This select sample of developed country population representative data on physical activity is not exhaustive, as there are hundreds of such studies in the literature. Furthermore, each country asks about physical activity prevalence in different ways. Some countries (specific data from Singapore, Japan and Australia appears in Table 3.1) ask about "exercise and structured aerobic physical activity," whereas other surveys ask more generic questions about moderate-intensity leisure time and other domains of physical activity, including England and the U.S. (Stamatakis et al., 2009; Carlson, Densmore, Fulton, Yore, & Kohl, 2008). For countries where "structured aerobic exercise" questions were asked, between a quarter and a third of all adults reach the 30 minutes of physical activity per day threshold, and in the countries where slightly more generic moderate-intensity physical activity questions were asked, the prevalence rates vary, typically from around 35% to 50% meeting the "sufficiently active" threshold (Table 3.1).

These national data all identify that the prevalence of physical inactivity (the risk factor) is high with between half and three quarters of adult populations not achieving sufficient physical activity for health. Moreover, physical inactivity is three to four times as prevalent in the population as tobacco smoking, and two to three times as prevalent as high blood pressure, high cholesterol, or obesity. Thus, physical inactivity is the most prevalent non-communicable

Table 3.1. Examples of population prevalence rates of "sufficiently active" for health (meeting physical activity recommendations).

Country/ year	Sample size (N)	Recommended level for "sufficiently active"	Population prevalence rate of "sufficiently active"
Singapore (2004)	4,084	30 mins	25%
Japan (Shibata, 2009)	1,932	Meet 23 MET hours/ week	28.3%
Health survey for England 2008	15,102	5 days x 30 mins	42% M, 31% F
Welsh Health Survey 2008	13,045	5 days/week	38% M, 22% F
United States CDC (JAMA, 2008)	Figures not available	Regular PA, 5 days 30 mins	49.7% M, 46.7% F
Canada (CFLRI, 2009)	7,601	30+ or more mins/day MVPA	48%
Australia National Health Survey 2007 (Australian Bureau of Statistics, 2008)	21,000	Not "sedentary/ low active" (based on regular exercise)	32% M, 24% F
Netherlands (Proper, 2006)	2,417 Dutch workers	30 mins/day	53.7%

Note: Physical activity measures differed by study; M=male; F=female; MET=multiple of resting energy expenditure (a measure of intensity of activity); PA=physical activity; MVPA=moderate-vigorous physical activity

disease risk factor, contributing to a percentage of the overall burden of disease and ill health (Bauman & Miller, 2004). Table 3.1 demonstrates that the physically inactive population fraction is high across all countries, highlighting that the public health need to increase physical activity is important for all adults.

The next component of a public health approach to physical inactivity is to describe the population-at-risk and potential solutions in more detail. Here, assessing the potential for dog walking requires an estimate of the rates of dog ownership or number of dogs in developed countries (Table 3.2). Since there is no accurate and standardized measure (e.g., Census) of the prevalence of dog ownership by country, these data can only be considered estimates. Much of this information is derived from pet food manufacturers or pet care associations, who estimate the number of dogs based on the amount of pet-related product sold in each country. In some countries estimates are provided for the total number of dogs, and for other countries it is the number of households that own a dog. The household-base estimate underestimates the potential health benefits from dog walking because each dog-owning household typically owns between 1 and 1.6 dogs (AVMA, 2006), and this ratio will vary by country.

The data in Table 3.2 show the total human populations and the approximate rates of dog ownership by country. Some countries such as the United States, France, Australia, and Sao Paolo Province in Brazil have high rates of dog ownership. In analyses at the household level, typically between one-sixth and one-third of the households has a dog. This provides an estimate of the population of dogs available for dog walking but does not give clear information of household composition, as the number of humans per household varies substantially between countries.

Prevalence and trends in dog walking in populations

Table 3.3 shows a selection of large scale studies from different countries that compared physical activity levels of dog owners and non-dog owners and assessed dog walking among dog owners. The studies were based on reasonably large samples, and covered populations from the United States, Canada, Australia, and Japan. There were different metrics used to assess physical activity and dog walking, but it can be seen that, in general, dog owners were slightly more active than non-dog owners (Coleman et al., 2008; Cutt et al., 2008c; Brown & Rhodes, 2006; Shibata, Oka, Harada, Nakamura, & Muraoka, 2009). For some studies, there was no difference between dog owner and non-dog owner physical activity (Bauman, Russell, Furber, & Dobson, 2001; Schofield & Mummery, 2005; Coleman et al., 2008; Thorpe et al., 2006). However, an important observation is that across studies, half or more of the dog owners did not report reaching recommended levels of physical activity. This is despite the observation that reaching the "150 minutes per week physical activity threshold" could be achieved through once-daily 25 minutes of dog walking.

There were too few studies examining the frequency of dog walking by household members, or the person-level analysis to determine who, in the household, was walking their dog(s). Furthermore, while many households reported at least some dog walking, these levels were often below that recom-

Table 3.2. Approximate rates of dog ownership or numbers of dogs by country.

Country	Approx. Human population in millions (2008) [Ω]	Dog ownership rates or estimated number of dogs
United Kingdom / England	59 M	6.1 M dogs in 2001, recent est. 8M dogs (2009); 24% households have a dog (Westgarth 2007)
United States	305 M	Ranged from 52.9M dogs in 1996 to 72-73 M dogs in 2005/6 (estimates as high as 77M dogs in 2006)[¶]; 42M dog owning households
Canada	32 M	Statcan estimate: 5.7 M dogs in 3.7M dog owning households
Japan	128 M	16-18% households have a dog; estimates range from 9.6-11M dogs
China	1325 M	Euromonitor International estimates ~22M dogs; some suggestion of an increase from 5% households in 1999 to 15% in 2004
European countries	Europe 728 M (Aut 8, Swe 9, Ger 82, Fra 60, Hun 10, Irl 4, Ita 58)	Austria ~0.5M dogs; Sweden ~0.8M dogs; Germany 13% households and 4.7-5M dogs; France 27% households and 8.8-9M dogs[¶]; Hungary 1.8M dogs; Ireland 35% households; Italy 4.5M households and 5.8-7M dogs Total Europe ~41M dogs, 21% of households
Australia	20 M	38% households have a dog; estimates range from 3.7-4M dogs [¶]
Central and South America	Brazil 195 M Costa Rica 4 M	Brazil ~27M dogs, one study showed 53% households in Sao Paulo had a dog[¶]; Costa Rica sample, around 50% households have a dog [¶]

Footnote: M=million; ¶ High dog: total population ratio

Data sources: U.S. pet ownership survey, 2007; pet food manufacturers / American Pet Product Association and American Pet Product Manufacturing Association Surveys, Pet Food Institute and dog food consumption-based national estimates; Census or national statistics collections; Sao Paulo data from Revista de Saude Publica, 2005:39:6.

[Ω] 2008 World Population data sheet, Population Reference Bureau (http://www.prb.org/publications/datasheets.aspx)

mended for health. However, some research has shown that people who walk their dogs every day were more likely to reach the recommended physical activity levels than those who did not walk their dogs (Cutt et al., 2008c; Coleman et al., 2008). A recent study of older adults with objectively assessed physical activity in the United Kingdom observed dog walking as a significant contributor to total walking (Harris, Owen, Victor, Adams, & Cook, 2009). Finally, some research suggests that acquiring a dog can increase physical activity time by 20 to 30 minutes per week of recreational walking (Cutt et al., 2008c).

Nonetheless, these data still clearly suggest that many dogs are walked infrequently, and that the majority of dog owners do no or little dog walking (Bauman et al., 2001). These results also have canine health implications. While no physical activity-related guidelines exist for canine health, once-daily walks are considered a minimum (Serpell, 1991).

There are very few data sets that can provide estimates of trends in dog walking. One such data set is the American Time Use data, where careful approaches to coding have created a variable called "dog walking"; this includes other dog-related care, such as veterinarian visits, but is likely to mostly capture time spent dog walking (Tudor-Locke et al., 2007; Tudor-Locke & Ham, 2008). Data from serial Time Use surveys suggests that walking the dog may have declined at the population level, from around 9.4% in 1985, to 5.4% in 1992-1994, and to 2.6% in 2003. The low 2003 population rate of dog walking of 2.6% of adult Americans was further examined (Tudor-Locke & Ham, 2008) and showed little variation by gender. Higher rates of dog walking were found among middle-aged compared with young or older adults, and among tertiary educated compared with high school education only. In 2003, Americans who walked their dogs did so for a median of 30 minutes, which is equivalent to the recommended level of physical activity for health benefit. This suggests that if dog owners can be encouraged to walk their dogs, it is likely this will, by itself, reach their daily physical activity goal for health.

These data are surprising for a number of reasons. First, there has been a likely increase in the total number of dogs in the U.S. during this period (see Table 3.2), suggesting that the rates of dog walking should have increased and not decreased. Second, there is evidence that human-dog interactions have moved from a predominantly "working relationship" in previous centuries, to a "companion-based" attachment (and a resultant sense of "dog obligation" [Brown & Rhodes, 2006]), and this would suggest that dog walking should have increased. In sum, these data provide indirect evidence that despite an increased canine population in the U.S., the level of dog walking has decreased.

Table 3.3. Prevalence of dog ownership, physical activity, and dog walking in studies across several countries.

Author (year of study, country)	Sample data (size, gender, % dog owners)	Mean minutes of total PA/ week	% achieving recommended level of PA	Mean minutes of total walking/week	Prevalence of dog walking	Mean mins DW/week	Mean frequency DW/week
Bauman et al. (2001) Australia	N=894; 45.6% male, 46% DO	DO: 210 NO: 198	DO: 46.9% NO: 47.3%	DO: 120 NO: 102	DO: 41%	DO: 57.0/ week	DO: 3.0
Schofield et al. (2004) Australia	N=1237; 57.3% DO	DO: 346.4 NO: 334.8	DO: 51.5% NO: 48.5%	*Walking for leisure* DO: 114.9 NO: 108.2	*By household member* DO: 60%	DO: 30.0/ walk (mode)	*By household member* DO: 7.0
Brown (2006) Canada	N=351; 50.4% male; 19.9% DO	DO: 410.3* NO: 287.5		DO: 300.2* NO: 168.4			
Cutt et al. (2008) Australia	N=1813; 40.5% male; 44% DO	DO: 322.4** NO: 267.1	DO: 61.2% NO: 54.1%	DO: 150.3** NO: 110.9	DO: 78%		DO: 2.6
Coleman et al. (2008) U.S.	N=2199; 52% male; 27.8% DO	*Objectively measured PA* DW: 35±25 NO: 33±24	DO: 46.9%* NO: 46.0%		DO: 70%	DO: 180±186	
Shibara & Oka (2009) Japan	N=5177; 50% male; 18% DO	*PA (METs-h/ wk):* DO: 17.0** NDO: 10.9	DO: 32.9% NO: 25.2%	*(METs-h/wk)* DO: 12.4* NO: 10.			

Yabroff (2008) U.S.	N=41514; 49% male; 17.7% DO		DO: 129.3* NO: 119.7
Ham & Epping (2006) U.S.	N=1282; 41% male; 100% DO		80.2% 1+ walks/day	42.3% 30 min or more/day
Thorpe et al. (2006) U.S.	N= 2533; adults 70-79yrs; 51.7% male; 12.9% DO	Any exercise % DO: 67.2 NPO: 64.0	walking DO: 67.9* NPO: 32.1

Legend: DO=dog owner, NO=non-dog owner, NPO=non-pet owners, PA=moderate-vigorous physical activity, METs-h/wk= metabolic equivalents hours/week; *P < .05, **P < .001, PA=physical activity, DW=dog walking

Barriers to physical activity: Lack of time and television viewing

The next step in a public health approach to increasing rates of physical activity is to describe why people say they are not physically active. Research into the most frequently reported physical activity barriers has identified a range of real and perceived personal and environmental factors that influence being physically active.

The physical environment may influence dog walking behaviors, but is also likely to influence walking in general without dogs. That is, dog owners appreciate the same environmental qualities for walking as non-dog owners (Cutt, Giles-Corti, Wood, Knuiman, & Burke, 2008a). Having access to large areas of attractive neighborhood public open space is important for walking (Cutt et al., 2008a; Sugiyama, Francis, Middleton, Owen, & Giles-Corti, 2010; Francis et al., 2010), and the number and location of parks are associated with physical activity (Cohen, McKenzie, Sehgal, Williamson, Golinelli, & Lurie, 2007; McKenzie et al., 2007). Other attributes such as connected streets, footpaths, destinations to walk to, and a safe neighborhood are also associated with more walking (Brownson, Baker, Housemann, Brennan, & Bacak, 2001). For example, in the United Kingdom, Jones et al. (2009) reported that residents in deprived areas had poorer perceived accessibility to green space and had safety concerns that limited their walking. Specifically for dog walking, a U.S. study found that women were 3.3 times more likely to walk a dog in the neighborhood if safety was average compared with below average (Suminski, Poston, Petosa, Stevens, & Katzenmoyer, 2005). While dog owners appear to appreciate the same qualities in parks as non-dog owners, they also desire parks with relevant dog-related infrastructure such as appropriate dog-related signage and dog litter removal bags (Cutt et al., 2008a, d). This suggests that dog owners may be encouraged to walk with their dogs more often if they have access to parks within their local area that support their presence.

In Western societies, "lack of time" is the most often cited reason why people are not (more) physically active. In a recent European-wide study of sport and physical activity from 27 countries (Eurobarometer, 2010, n=27,000 adults), 45% of reported that "I do not have time" as the leading reason for not being physically active. Other reasons were less frequently reported, and comprised (i) having a disability or illness (reported by 13%); (ii) don't like exercise (7%); (iii) too expensive (5%); (iv) no suitable sports facilities (3%); and (v) having no-one to exercise with (3%).

In Australian studies, up to 73% of younger adults report lack of time as a barrier to physical activity (Welch, McNaughton, Hunter, Hume, & Crawford, 2009), followed by lack of motivation, and childcare responsibilities, and for older adults, poor health and injury were the most prevalent (Booth, Owen, Bauman, Clavisi, & Leslie, 2000). In a rural U.S. female sample, the most frequent reasons were "lack of time," no motivation or interest, and not having anyone to exercise with (Osuji, Lovegreen, Elliott, & Brownson, 2006). In another U.S. female sample, almost a third (30%) reported lack of time as a barrier, although lack of willpower and lack of support were also frequent responses (Rye, Rye, Tessaro, & Coffindaffer, 2009).

Reported "lack of time" or being "too busy" is more likely to be an attribution or excuse for not being active. This is evidenced by a closer examination of adults' time use patterns in developed countries. For many, sedentary behaviors emerge as the most common leisure-time activities, with television watching and Internet use as the leading passive forms of recreation. To demonstrate this further, Table 3.4 highlights the prevalence of television watching and other forms of electronic recreation time in different countries. Most show that adults and adolescents spend at least two hours a day in these sedentary activities. These data come from national Time Use studies and several from large population-based cohort studies. The highest television watching prevalence rates are from Scotland and England: the former at over three hours a day, but this includes other screen-based entertainment as well as television watching; the latter (Jakes et al., 2003) at over 21 hours per week (over three hours a day) for television watching alone. Similar rates of screen time are seen among adolescents in the U.S. and in Europe (Currie, 2008; YRBS, 2009).

Thus, the most frequent reason for not being active ("no time") is cited, despite people watching television and other sedentary activities for an average of two to three hours daily. There may be other climate, safety, and environmental barriers, but for the majority of these television watchers, this is discretionary time that *could* be spent being physically active. Among dog owners, replacing only a quarter of their sedentary screen time at home with dog walking would achieve their daily physical activity needs for health.

Theoretical reasons why dog walking is appropriate as a physical activity strategy for whole populations

There are a large number of dogs (and households with a dog) available for walking, making this a physical activity strategy with potential population-wide reach. In addition, a public health approach to physical activity requires that there are theoretically sound behavior-change reasons why dog walking might provide a good opportunity for increasing physical activity.

Table 3.4. Television watching prevalence across different countries (selected countries, representative samples, self-report television hours). (Shaded rows are adolescent data.)

Country	N	Measures	Median/% of population	Reference
European youth, aged 11–15 years	~ 3,000 sampled in 41 countries	Reported TV watching > 2 hours	2/3 of European adolescents watch ≥2hrs/day	HBSC report 2005/2006, Inequalities in young people's health, WHO Europe 2008 (41 country study, Currie 2008)
U.S. adolescents	14,103	Reported TV watching > 3hours/day	35.4 % of adolescents	Youth Risk behavior survey 2007
U.S. adults	13,100	Watching TV	3.2 hrs/weekday; 4.0 hrs/weekends	American Time Use Survey 2009 (US Department of Labor 2010)
Australian adults	3,900	Audio/visual activities	16.3 hrs/week;	Australian Bureau of Statistics 2008 – from 2006 Time Use Survey AusDiab study (Dunstan 2010)
	8,800	TV watching per day	approx 2 hrs/day	
United Kingdom adults	4,941	TV & Video/ DVDs, radio, listen to music	2.3 hours/day	UK 2006, from Time Use Study 2005 (Note: NOP 2005 reports 18hrs/week of TV alone)
Scottish adults	7,940	TV/screen-based media	Over 3hrs/day	Scottish Health Survey 2003 (Stamatakis et al 2009)

English adults	14,189	TV viewing	21.2 hrs/wk (M) 21.9 hrs/wk (F)	EPIC-Norfolk population-based study (Jakes et al 2003)
Canadian adults	19,597	Watching TV	2.1 Hours per day	Statistics Canada, 2005 General Social Survey, Time Use (NOP survey 2005: 14.7 hrs/week)
European adults 15 EC countries	Population data	TV watching	Median by 2005 was 200 mins/day	Vergeer et al in Konig, Nelissen and Huysmans 2009
Asian countries, adults	30,000 in 30 countries	TV viewing time per week	Japan 17.9 hrs/week, Taiwan 18.9 hrs/week, Philippines 21 hrs, Thailand 22.4 hrs	NOP World Culture Survey 2005 (Note: the global mean=16.6 hours TV watched/week, average non work internet time estimated at 9 hours/week)

Legend: M=males; F=females

Behavioral theories are useful because they can explain "why people are or are not physically active." One commonly used theoretical formulation is social learning theory, also known as social cognitive theory (Bandura, 2004). This theory has a number of elements, but the key components include (i) the preventive behavior is accessible to those at risk; (ii) increasing people's confidence makes a behavior more likely; and (iii) performing the behavior is reinforcing and cues cognitive and affective responses that lead to repetition of the behavior (Glanz, Rimer, & Viswanath, 2008). Other theories including the Diffusion of Innovations (Bauman et al., 2006) framework have examined why people adopt and maintain new behaviors. Important components include that (i) behaviors are easy to perform; (ii) that they can be trialed initially to see if people enjoy them; (iii) that they can fit into people's lifestyles and schedules; and (iv) that they confer advantages to people over other ways of doing the same thing or other ways of spending their time. A third theoretical framework is the Theory of Reasoned Action (Theory of Planned Behavior) (Glanz et al., 2008). Here the determinants of behavior start with the (i) prevailing social norms about a behavior; (ii) adopting particular sets of beliefs and values about the behavior; and (iii) confidence in performing the behavior. All these lead to intention to carry out the behavior, and in turn intention predicts behavior.

These three theoretical formulations all fit very well in describing the intrapersonal determinants of dog walking. The behavior of dog walking is strongly related to all of these theoretical attributes, including being an accessible behavior, easy to do, confidence enhancing, behaviorally reinforcing, trialable, can have flexible timing, and is theoretically an advantageous way of starting and maintaining physical activity compared with more complex structured exercise. It can be adopted at all ages and potentially by all population groups. At the individual behavioral level, dog walking meets all the theoretical criteria for an optimal population-wide approach to increasing physical activity.

There are also individual and dog-specific correlates of dog walking. "Dog obligation," or the sense of responsibility to walk a dog daily, is an important correlate of dog walking intention and behavior (Cutt, Giles-Corti, & Knuiman, 2008d; Christian, Giles-Corti, & Knuiman, 2010; Brown & Rhodes, 2006). However most are individual-level cognitive-behavioral theories, and in addition we need to consider the social and physical environments in which physical activity might occur. Whether people will walk their dogs is also determined by their social environment, community safety, and perceptions of whether others like them are walking their dogs. Social support has been shown to be an important predictor of physical activity (Giles-Corti & Donovan, 2003; Pan et al., 2009). For example, people with a low level of perceived social support from their family, friends, school, or the workplace are twice as likely to be sedentary (Stahl et al., 2001). The family dog is likely to be an understated but important form of social support that could potentially facilitate and reinforce walking behavior (McNicholas & Collis, 2000). Ball et al. (2001) found that women who reported no company or pet to walk with were 31% less likely to walk for exercise or recreation. In addition, walking with a dog can provide owners with a greater feeling of safety, particularly when walking at night or in an unsafe neighborhood (Serpell, 1991; Raymore & Scott, 1998). In addition, aspects of the physical environment including well-maintained sidewalks, places such as trails and parks to use and to walk to, and safe communities are all aspects of the physical environment that are also highly relevant to dog walking. Use of green space and environmental facilities is more likely among dog owners, suggesting that dog owners are an important user group that need to be considered in the design and allocation of parks and other local facilities (Schipperijn, Stigsdotter, Randrup, & Troelsen, 2010).

Approaches to increasing dog walking

Dog walking has the potential to become one of the most effective ways to increase community levels of walking (Voelker, 2006). A population-wide health impact would result from increases in dog walking. As there are many households with dogs, and walking with a dog is achievable by all age groups, the population health potential of dog walking is substantial.

To date, few community-wide efforts have been carried out that have included dog walking as a central strategy, despite its theoretical and conceptual advantages, and population reach. A few community-wide or national social marketing efforts to promote physical activity have used dog walking in their mass media messages, as examples of realistic, achievable, and regular physical activity. Several large scale mass media campaigns in particular have had dog walking messages. Examples include the Push Play national campaign in New Zealand in 2002-2006 and the Western Australian "Find 30" campaign (Bauman et al., 2003; Find 30 campaign, 2010). Mass communications are a central platform of wide-scale strategies to encourage physical activity, and it should be a centerpiece of community-wide campaigns and public health programs to target householders with messages and a call to action to increase dog walking. Most dog owners know they should walk their dog regularly, and engaging with this sense of "obligation" (Brown & Rhodes, 2006), this strategy could influence their attitudes to dog walking, inform them of the relationship to achieving physical activity recommendations, and catalyze behavioral trialing for those who do not walk their dogs at all.

Other approaches to dog walking interventions have used volunteer or convenient samples, or targeted special population sub-groups. Specific programs may target dog owners, or even target those without a dog to trial dog walking, for example, using shelter dogs. These interventions may be effective in influencing specific at-risk groups, but are using small sample sizes, and are less likely to have a whole population effect (Johnson & Meadows, 2010; Kushner, Blatner, Jewell, & Rudloff, 2006).

Health benefits that would accrue if population dog walking increased

The health benefits of population dog walking was estimated by analyzing real population physical activity data to model the effects of increasing (dog) walking on the proportion of the population reaching the "recommended" levels of physical activity for health benefit. Actual data from a national (Active Australia) survey were used, and a hypothetical baseline rate of "35% sufficiently active" was used (Figure 3.1). Since the prevalence of dog ownership is between one-sixth and one-third of the population, both of these fractions were used. In this simulation, it was assumed that all dog owners would increase their dog walking. As shown in Figure 3.1, if all dog owners added 60 minutes of dog walking per week to their current levels of physical activity, it would increase the "sufficiently active" rates by 5% to 10% (depending on population dog ownership rates). Further benefits would accrue if 90 minutes of dog walking were added to current physical activity levels. The greatest beneficial shifts would accrue if "insufficiently active" people began dog walking and increased their walking by 60 or 90 minutes per week. For example, if one third of inactive people increased their dog walking by 90 minutes per week, this would result in 60% of this population being "sufficiently active" (Figure 3.1).

Given fixed relative risks of disease in relation to physical activity (Bauman & Miller, 2004; USDHHS, 2008), and the population prevalence changes in physical activity that would result from increased dog walking, we can directly estimate health benefits. The best case scenario is "to increase weekly dog walking by 90 minutes" among the inactive, resulting in 60% sufficiently active (an absolute increase of 25% in the population prevalence from 35% at baseline). Applying the concept of population attributable risk (Bauman & Miller, 2004), we can calculate that this increase in walking as a result of walking the dog would prevent 12% of all new and fatal cases of coronary

Figure 3.1. Synthetic modeling: effects of weekly increases in dog walking time on population rates of "sufficient physically active."

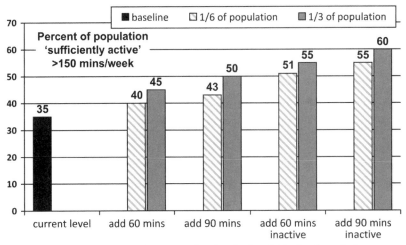

artery disease, prevent the onset of 9% of new diabetes cases, and reduce the incidence of colon cancer, falls in the elderly, stroke, and anxiety/depression by 5% to 10% in the population. The health savings that would accrue from this increase in dog walking would be many billions of dollars. In addition, the non-quantified benefits in terms of community well-being, functional status gains in the elderly, and improvements in social connections would provide a very significant contribution to improving the quality of life of our communities.

Conclusion

Dog walking has the potential to confer human health benefits through increases in physical activity. Given the high prevalence of dog owners worldwide, this effect would be larger than any physical activity intervention examined to date. Furthermore, this kind of intervention has several potential benefits. First, dog walking could possibly play a role in primary and secondary prevention of chronic diseases, improve mental health, and provide social support. Dog walking can also impact an individual's social environment. As it relates to the canine, walking may reduce and/or delay obesity and obesity-related problems in dogs (Bland, Guthrie-Jones, Taylor, & Hill, 2009; German, 2006) as well as enhance musculoskeletal health. Canine obesity is often related to the body mass index of their owners, so dog walking may have benefits for both owner and dog (Nijland, Stam, & Seidell, 2009).

There are several challenges and opportunities suggested by this public health approach to increasing physical activity. First, dog walking should be encouraged in community physical activity programs and should be more vigorously supported as an intervention component. Specific communications strategies targeting dog owners would be a generic and important start. Second, and more confronting, is the scale of change required to improve population health. Influencing only a few dog owners will not impact population health. Current intervention efforts to encourage dog walking usually target small volunteer samples or special groups; while these programs will help those exposed to them, they will not impact community physical activity levels and population health unless they are made more generalizable and have wider population reach.

In conclusion, dog owners are a large population target, and many dogs are insufficiently walked. There is great public health potential for dogs to become an effective physical activity strategy for human health, but there are major challenges in reaching the many millions of insufficiently active dog owners worldwide. These challenges include the perceptions and low motivation of many dog owners regarding dog walking, the lack of urban environments to walk dogs, and issues around the frequency and duration amount that dogs are actually walked. When dog walking is perceived as a feasible, affordable, and regular solution to an increasingly sedentary population, then it may start to have a public health impact.

References

Australian Bureau of Statistics. (2008). *4153.0-How Australians use their time, 2006.* Canberra. Retrieved from http://www.abs.gov.au/AUSSTATS/abs@.nsf/Loo kup/4153.0Main+Features12006?OpenDocument

Australian Bureau of Statistics. (2008). *4364.0-National health survey: summary of results, 2007-2008.* Canberra. Retrieved from http://www.abs.gov.au/ausstats/abs@.nsf/mf/4364.0

AVMA. (2006). Household pet ownership and by selected characteristic. *American Veterinary Medical Association, Schaumburg, IL, U.S. pet ownership and demographics sourcebook*, 1993 & 1997. Retrieved from http://www.allcountries.org/uscensus/424_household_pet_ownership_and_by_selected.html

Ball, K., Bauman, A., Leslie, E., & Owen, N. (2001). Perceived environmental aesthetics and convenience and company are associated with walking for exercise among Australian adults. *Preventive Medicine, 33*(5), 434-440.

Bandura, A. (2004). Health promotion by social cognitive means. *Health Education & Behavior, 31*(2), 143-164.

Bauman, A. E., Russell, S. J., Furber, S. E., & Dobson, A. J. (2001). The epidemiology of dog walking: An unmet need for human and canine health. *Medical Journal of Australia, 175*(11-12), 632-634.

Bauman, A., Bellew, B., Vita, P., Brown, W., & Owen, N. (2002). Getting Australia active: towards better practice for the promotion of physical activity. *National Public Health Partnership*. Melbourne, Australia, March, 2002. ISBN: 0-9580326-2-9.

Bauman, A., McLean, G., Hurdle, D., Walker, S., Boyd, J., van Aalst, I., & Carr, H. (2003). Evaluation of the national 'Push Play' campaign in New Zealand—creating population awareness of physical activity. *New Zealand Medical Journal* (Original articles 8th August 2003), 116, 1179.

Bauman, A., & Miller, Y. (2004). The public health potential of health enhancing physical activity (HEPA). In P. Oja & J. Borms (Eds.), *Multidisciplinary perspectives of physical education and sport science* (pp. 125-149). Oxford, UK: Meyer and Meyer Sport Publishers.

Bauman, A. E., Nelson, D. E., Pratt, M., Matsudo, V., & Schoeppe, S. (2006). Dissemination of physical activity evidence, programs, policies, and surveillance in the international public health arena. *American Journal of Preventive Medicine*, (4 Suppl), 57-65.

Bauman, A., Allman-Farinelli, M., Huxley, R., & James, W. P. T. (2008). Leisure-time physical activity alone may not be a sufficient public health approach to prevent obesity—a focus on China. *Obesity Reviews*, 9 (Suppl. 1), 119–126.

Bland, I. M., Guthrie-Jones, A., Taylor, R. D., & Hill, J. (2010). Dog obesity: Veterinary practices' and owners' opinions on cause and management. *Preventive Veterinary Medicine, 94*, 310-315.

Booth, M. L., Owen, N., Bauman, A., Clavisi, O., & Leslie, E. (2000). Social, cognitive and perceived environment influences associated with physical activity in older Australians. *Preventive Medicine, 31*, 15-22.

Brown, S. G., & Rhodes, R. E. (2006). Relationships among dog ownership and leisure-time walking in western Canadian adults. *American Journal of Preventive Medicine, 30*, 131-136.

Brownson, R. C., Baker, E. A., Housemann, R. A., Brennan, L. K., & Bacak, S. J. (2001). Environmental and policy determinants of physical activity in the United States. *American Journal of Public Health, 91*, 1995-2003.

Carlson, S. A., Densmore, D., Fulton, J. E., Yore, M. M., & Kohl, H. W. 3rd. (2009). Differences in physical activity prevalence and trends from 3 U.S. surveillance systems: NHIS, NHANES, and BRFSS. *Journal of Physical Activity and Health, 6,* S18-27.

Centers for Disease Control and Prevention (CDC). (2008). Prevalence of regular physical activity among adults United States 2001 and 2005. *Journal of American Medical Association. 299,* 30-32.

CFLRI 2009. Canadian Fitness and Lifestyle Research Institute, physical activity levels of adult Canadians. Retrieved from http://www.cflri.ca/eng/statistics/su rveys/2008PhysicalActivityMonitor.php

Chau, J., Bonfiglioli, C., Chey, T., & Bauman, A. (2009). The Cinderella of public health news: Physical activity coverage in Australian newspapers, 1986-2006. *Australian and New Zealand Journal of Public Health, 33,*189-92.

Christian, H., Giles-Corti, B., & Knuiman, M. (2010). 'I'm just a'-walking the dog.' correlates of regular dog walking. *Family & Community Health, 33,* 44-52.

Coleman, K. J., Rosenberg, D. E, Conway, T. L., Sallis, J. F., Saelens, B. E., Frank, L. D., & Cain, K. (2008). Physical activity, weight status, and neighborhood characteristics of dog walkers. *Preventive Medicine, 47,* 309-312.

Cohen, D. A., McKenzie, T. L., Sehgal, A., Williamson, S., Golinelli, D., & Lurie, N. (2007). Contribution of public parks to physical activity. *American Journal of Public Health, 7,* 509-514.

Currie, C. (Ed.). (2008). Inequalities in young people's health: Health behaviour in school-aged children. International Report from the 2005/2006 HBSC Survey. World Health Organization Regional Office for Europe, Copenhagen, Denmark.

Cutt, H., Giles-Corti, B., & Knuiman M. (2007). Dog ownership, health and physical activity: A critical review of the literature. *Health & Place, 13,* 261-272.

Cutt, H. E., Giles-Corti, B., Wood, L. J., Knuiman M. W., & Burke V. (2008a). Barriers and motivators for owners walking their dog: Results from qualitative research. *Health Promotion Journal of Australia, 19,* 118-124.

Cutt, H. E, Knuiman, M. W., & Giles-Corti, B. (2008b). Does getting a dog increase recreational walking? *International Journal of Behavior Nutrition and Physical Activity, 5,* 17.

Cutt, H., Giles-Corti, B., Knuiman, M., Timperio, A., & Bull, F. (2008c). Understanding dog owners' increased levels of physical activity: results from RESIDE. *American Journal of Public Health, 98,* 66-69.

Cutt, H., Giles-Corti B., & Knuiman, M. (2008d). Encouraging physical activity through dog walking: Why don't some owners walk with their dog? *Preventive Medicine, 46,* 120-126.

Dunstan, D. W., Barr, E. L., Healy, G. N., Salmon, J., Shaw, J. E., Balkau, B., Magliano, D. J., Cameron, A. J., Zimmet, P. Z., & Owen N. (2010). Television viewing time and mortality: The Australian Diabetes, Obesity and Lifestyle Study (AusDiab). *Circulation, 121*, 384-391.

Eurobarometer Survey, Special EB 334 / Wave 72.3-TNS Opinion & Social. (2010). Sport and physical activity. Directorate-General Education and Culture, European Commission, Brussels. Retrieved from http://ec.europa.eu/public_opinion/archives/ebs/ebs_334_en.pdf

Find 30 Campaign, Heart Foundation of Western Australia, Perth WA. (2010). Retrieved from http://www.findthirtyeveryday.com.au/

German, A. J. (2006). The growing problem of obesity in dogs and cats. *Journal of Nutrition, 136*, 1940S-1946S.

Glanz, K., Rimer, B., & Viswanath, K. (Eds). (2008). *Health behavior and health education: Theory, research, and practice, 4th ed.* New Jersey: Jossey-Bass.

Giles-Corti, B., & Donovan, R. J. (2003). Increasing walking: Relative influences of individual, social environmental, and physical environmental correlates of walking. *American Journal of Public Health, 93*, 1583-1589.

Ham, S. A., & Epping, J. (2006). Dog walking and physical activity in the United States. *Preventing Chronic Disease, 3*, A47.

Harris, T. J., Owen, C. G., Victor, C. R., Adams, R., & Cook, D.G. (2009). What factors are associated with physical activity in older people, assessed objectively by accelerometry? *British Journal of Sports Medicine, 43*, 442-450.

Haskell, W. L., Lee, I-M., Pate, R. R., Powell, K. E., Blair, S. N., Franklin, B. A., Macera, C. A., Heath, G. W., Thompson, P. D., & Bauman, A. (2007). Physical activity and public health: Updated recommendation for adults from the American College of Sports Medicine and the American Heart Association. *Medicine Science and Sports Exercise, 39*, 1423-1434.

Health Survey for England—2008: Physical activity and fitness. (2009). *National Health Service.* Retrieved from http://www.ic.nhs.uk/statistics-and-data-collections/health-and-lifestyles-related-surveys/health-survey-for-england/health-survey-for-england--2008-physical-activity-and-fitness

Jakes, R. W., Day, N. E., Khaw, K. T., Luben, R., Oakes, S., Welch, A., Bingham, S., & Wareham, N. J. (2003). Television viewing and low participation in vigorous recreation are independently associated with obesity and markers of cardiovascular disease risk: EPIC-Norfolk population-based study. *European Journal of Clinical Nutrition, 57*, 1089–1096.

Johnson, R.A, & Meadows, R.T. (2010). Dog-Walking: Motivation for adherence to a walking program. *Clinical Nurse Research, 19*(4), 387-402. DOI:10.1177/1054773810373122.

Jones, A., Hillsdon, M., & Coombes, E. (2009). Greenspace access, use, and physical activity: understanding the effects of area deprivation. *Preventive Medicine, 49*, 500-505.

Kushner, R. F., Blatner D. J., Jewell, D.E., & Rudloff, K. (2006). The PPET Study: People and pets exercising together. *Obesity, 14*, 1762-1770.

McNicholas, J., & Collis, G. M. (2000). Dogs as catalysts for social interactions: Robustness of the effect. *British Journal of Psychology, 91*, 61-70.

Nelson, M. E., Rejeski, W. J., Blair, S. N., Duncan, P. W., Judge, J. O., King, A. C., Macera, C. A., Castaneda-Sceppa, C., American College of Sports Medicine & American Heart Association. (2007). Physical activity and public health in older adults: Recommendation from the American College of Sports Medicine and the American Heart Association. *Circulation, 116*, 1094-1105

Nijland, M. L., Stam, F., & Seidell, J.C. (2009). Overweight in dogs, but not in cats, is related to overweight in their owners. *Public Health Nutrition, 13*, 102-106.

NOP World Culture Survey. (2005). Global media habits. (Market research consortia data.) Retrieved from http://www.marketresearchworld.net/index.php?option=com_content&task=view&id=102

Owen, C. G., Nightingale, C. M., Rudnicka, A. R., Ekelund, U., McMinn, A. M., van Sluijs, E. M., Griffin, S. J., Cook, D. G., & Whincup, P. H. (2010). Family dog ownership and levels of physical activity in childhood: Findings from The Child Heart and Health Study in England. *American Journal of Public Health, 100*, 1669-1671.

Osuji, T., Lovegreen, S. L., Elliott, M., & Brownson, R. C. (2006). Barriers to physical activity among women in the rural midwest. *Women's Health, 44*, 41-55.

Pan, S., Cameron, C., DesMeules, M., Morrison, H., Craig, C.L., & Jiang, X. (2009). Individual, social, environmental, and physical environmental correlates with physical activity among Canadians: a cross-sectional study. *BMC Public Health, 9*, 21. DOI:10.1186/1471-2458-9-21.

Proper, K. I., & Hildebrandt, V. H. (2006). Physical activity among Dutch workers—differences between occupations. *Preventive Medicine, 43*, 42-45.

Raymore, L., & Scott, D. (1998). The characteristics and activities of older visitors to a metropolitan park district. *Journal of Park and Recreation Administration, 16*, 1-21.

Rye, J. A., Rye, S. L., Tessaro, I., & Coffindaffer, J. (2009). Perceived barriers to physical activity according to stage of change and body mass index in the West Virginia Wisewoman population. *Women's Health Issues, 19*, 126-134.

Schipperijn, J., Stigsdotter, U. K., Randrup, T., & Troelsen, J. (2010). Influences on the use of urban green space—a case study in Odense, Denmark. *Urban Forestry & Urban Greening, 9*, 25-32.

Schofield, G., Mummery, K., & Steel R. (2005). Dog ownership and human health-related physical activity: An epidemiological study. *Health Promotion Journal of Australia, 16*, 15-19.

Serpell, J. (1991). Beneficial effects of pet ownership on some aspects of human health and behaviour. *Journal of the Royal Society of Medicine, 84*, 717-720.

Shibata, A., Oka, K., Harada, K., Nakamura, Y., & Muraoka, I. (2009). Psychological, social, and environmental factors to meeting physical activity recommendations among Japanese adults. *International Journal of Behavioral Nutrition and Physical Activity, 6*, 60.

Stahl, T., Rutten, A., Nutbeam, D., Bauman, A., Kannas, L., Abel, T., Luschen, G. Rodriquez, D. J. A., Vinck, J., & van der Zee, J. (2001). The importance of the social environment for physically active lifestyle—results from an international study. *Social Science and Medicine, 5*, 1-10.

Stamatakis, E., Hamer, M., & Lawlor, D. A. (2009). Physical activity, mortality, and cardiovascular disease: Is domestic physical activity beneficial? The Scottish Health Survey—1995, 1998, and 2003. *American Journal of Epidemiology, 169*, 1191-1200.

Stamatakis, E., Hillsdon, M., Mishra, G., Hamer, M., & Marmot, M. (2009). Television viewing and other screen-based entertainment in relation to multiple socioeconomic status indicators and area deprivation: The Scottish Health Survey 2003. *Journal of Epidemiology and Community Health, 63*, 734-740.

Statistics Canada. (2005). *General Social Survey*. Ottawa. Retrieved from http://www.statcan.gc.ca/pub/12f0080x/2006001/t/4058341-eng.htm

Statistics Singapore. (2005). *National Health Survey 2004*. Singapore: Retrieved from http://www.singstat.gov.sg/pubn/papers/people/ssnsep05-pg19-20.pdf

Sugiyama, T., Francis, J., Middleton, N. J., Owen, N., & Giles-Corti, B. (2010). Associations between recreational walking and attractiveness, size, and proximity of neighborhood open spaces. *American Journal of Public Health, 100*, 1752-1757.

Suminski, R. R., Poston, W. S. C., Petosa, R. L, Stevens, E., & Katzenmoyer, L. M. (2005). Features of the neighborhood environment and walking by US adults. *American Journal of Preventive Medicine, 28*, 149-155.

Thorpe, R., Simonsick, E., Brach, J. S, Ayonayon, H., Satterfield, S., Harris, T. B., Garcia, M., & Kritchevsky, S. B. (2006). Dog ownership, walking behavior, and maintained mobility in late life. *Journal of the American Geriatric Society, 54*, 1419-1424.

Timperio, A., J. Salmon, Chu, B, Veitch, J. (2008). Is dog ownership or dog walking associated with weight status in children and their parents? *Health Promotion Journal of Australia, 19*, 60-63.

Tudor-Locke, C., & Ham, S. A. (2008). Walking behaviors reported in the American Time Use Survey 2003-2005. *Journal of Physical Activity and Health, 5*, 633-647.

Tudor-Locke, C., van der Ploeg, H. P., Bowles, H., Bittman, M., Fisher, K., Merom, D., Gershuny, J., Bauman, A., & Egerton, M. (2007). Walking behaviors from the 1965-2003 American Heritage Time Use Study (AHTUS). *International journal of Behavioral Nutrition and Physical Activity, 4*, 45.

U.K. National Statistics. (2006). *The Time Use Study, 2005.* London: Retrieved from http://www.statistics.gov.uk/articles/nojournal/time_use_2005.pdf

U.S. Department of Health and Human Services (USDHHS). (2008). *Physical activity guidelines for Americans.* Washington D.C.: US Department of Health and Human Services.

U.S. Department of Labor. (2010). *American Time Use Survey (ATUS).* Washington, DC: Retrieved from http://www.bls.gov/tus

Vergeer, M., Coenders, M., & Scheepers, P. (2009). Time spent on television in European countries: cross-national comparisons and explanations. Chapter 5. In R. Konig, P. Nelissen, & F. Huysmans (Eds.), *Meaningful media: Communication research on the social construction of reality.* Nijmegen, Netherlands: Tandem Felix Publishers.

Voelker, R. (2006). Studies suggest dog walking a good strategy for fostering fitness. *Journal of the American Medical Association, 296*, 643.

Welch, N., McNaughton, S. A., Hunter, W., Hume, C., Crawford, D. (2009). Is the perception of time pressure a barrier to healthy eating and physical activity among women? *Public Health Nutrition, 12*, 888-895.

Welsh Assembly Government. Cardiff. (2009). *Welsh Health Survey 2008: Initial Headline Results.* Retrieved from http://wales.gov.uk/docs/statistics/2009/090521sdr712009en.pdf

Westgarth, C., Pinchbeck, G. L., Bradshaw, J. W. S., Dawson, S., Gaskell, R. M., & Christley, R. M. (2007). Factors associated with dog ownership and contact with dogs in a UK community. *BMC Veterinary Research, 3*, 5.

WHO. (2009). *Global health risks: mortality and burden of disease attributable to selected major risks.* World Health Organization: Geneva. Retrieved from http://www.who.int/healthinfo/global_burden_disease/global_health_risks/en/index.html

WHO. (2010). *Global physical activity recommendations.* World Health Organization: Geneva. Retrieved from http://www.who.int/dietphysicalactivity/factsheet_recommendations/en/index.html

Wood, L., Giles-Corti, B., & Bulsara, M. (2005). The pet connection: Pets as a conduit for social capital? *Social Science & Medicine, 61*, 1159-1173.

Yabroff, K. R., Troiano, R. P., & Berrigan, D. (2008). Walking the dog: Is pet ownership associated with physical activity in California? *Journal of Physical Activity & Health, 5*, 216-228.

YRBS (2009). *Youth Risk Behavior Surveillance System*, U.S.Centers for Disease Control and Prevention. Reported in *MMWR* 2010; 59, SS-5, CDC Atlanta, GA. Retrieved from http://www.cdc.gov/HealthyYouth/yrbs/index.htm

Chapter 4

Dog walking as a catalyst for strengthening the social fabric of the community

Lisa L. Wood and Hayley E. Christian

"Social capital is the social glue, the weft and warp of the social fabric which comprises a myriad of interactions that make up our public and private lives."

(Eva Cox, Boyer lecture, 1995)

Pets and the social realm

Dogs and other pets are often widely regarded by their owners as social companions, and there is now considerable research documenting the role companion animals can play in providing companionship, social support, and alleviation of loneliness (Beck & Katcher, 2003; Katcher & Beck, 1983). While companionship and social support do appear in some of the dog walking research, this is primarily in reference to the role of dogs themselves in providing company and a motivation for their owners to walk (Cutt, Giles-Corti, Knuiman, & Burke, 2007). The focus of this chapter is the contribution dogs make to the broader social fabric of a community when they are out being walked. Anecdotally, many a dog owner will bear testimony to the occurrence of social interactions with other humans while out walking their dog, but to date there are only a small number of research studies to examine this phenomenon. Even less researched are the potential accumulated social benefits at the community level of having more people out and about walking their dogs.

The role of pets as social lubricants has been examined in two different studies undertaken at The University of Western Australia. The first was a study investigating the relationship between neighborhood design, social capital, and health; the study was broadly interested in identifying aspects of community that facilitate or hinder social capital formation (Wood, 2006). In focus groups, a number of participants mentioned interacting with neighbors as a result of a dog or other pet. Pet owners were 74% more likely to have a high social capital score than non-pet owners on a social capital scale (measuring trust, reciprocity, civic engagement, perceived friendliness, and social networks) after controlling for various demographic factors (Wood, Giles-Corti, & Bulsara, 2005).

The second study to explore the role of dogs as social facilitators was Cutt's Dogs and Physical Activity (DAPA) study, which examined the relationship between dog ownership and physical activity, in particular walking (Christian (née Cutt), Giles-Corti, & Knuiman, 2010; Cutt, Giles-Corti, & Knuiman, 2008; Cutt et al., 2007; Cutt, Giles-Corti, Knuiman, & Pikora, 2008; Cutt, Knuiman, & Giles-Corti, 2008). The study included both qualitative data (focus groups with dog owners and local government employees) and a survey of residents living in new residential estates (including dog and non-dog owners). The DAPA study investigated the amount of physical activity people undertake with their dog and dog-specific individual and environmental factors affecting people walking with their dog. While the main study results relate to correlates of physical activity and dog walking, some interesting findings also emerged in relation to the social dimension of dog walking, including interactions with other dog walkers.

These two studies highlight the potential role played by dogs and dog walking in fostering the social fabric of communities—the theme of this chapter. The chapter reviews and comments on the scattered but growing body of research and community interest in the role of companion animals (and particularly dogs) as facilitators of social interactions and sense of community within neighborhoods and communities, both among those who own dogs and the broader community. We have sought to synthesize the relevant published literature to date, interwoven with findings from qualitative and quantitative research undertaken over the last eight years at The University of Western Australia.

How does dog walking contribute to the social fabric of communities?

While pets have often been described as a bridge between humans and nature (Podberscek, 2000), there is an emerging body of evidence pointing to the way in which companion animals can also act as a social bridge between people, and further, contribute to the "ties that bind" communities together as a civil society (Wood, 2010). In drawing on the literature in this area and the research undertaken with colleagues in Western Australia, we identify six possible mechanisms through which dogs and dog walking can impact the social realm of communities. These are depicted in the following diagram and described in the sections that follow.

Figure 4.1. Dog walking contributes to the social realm of communities.

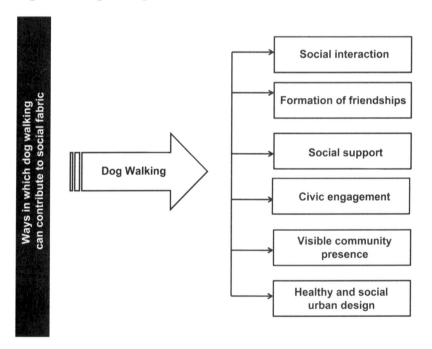

Social interaction

Before turning to the role of dogs as facilitators of social interaction, it is pertinent to consider social interaction in its broader sociological context. Humans are fundamentally social beings, yet there are concerns that the "harried isolating nature of modern life appears to be minimizing our capacity for human contact" (Walljasper, 2007, p. 10). While there is considerable evidence showing the health and well-being benefits of social ties, social networks, and social support (Berkman & Glass, 2000), the significance of informal and incidental forms of social interaction should not be discounted. Feeling a sense of connectedness to others within our proximity is said to be psychologically beneficial; relationships between neighbors and fellow community members need not be as close friends, but can valuably include acquaintances and people whom we can enjoy a chat with even if this merely takes the form of an informal chat (Albery, 2001). Moreover, the willingness of strangers to acknowledge or interact with each other can be viewed as a marker of sense of community and trust (Wood, 2006).

Although the term social interaction is more typically equated with conversation and verbal communication, there are numerous situations where humans interact with others in the absence of a spoken word. An interesting paradox arises in relation to social interaction among strangers in public settings. While the friendliness of residents to each other and to strangers can be viewed as a positive marker of sense of community, it has also been argued that in the highly individualized context of modern society, "everyday civility requires that strangers maintain a sense of separateness in crowded places" (Wise, 2008, p. 10) . Civil inattention is a term coined by Erving Goffman in the early 1960s to describe the behavioral rituals of self containment that people often invoke when encountering strangers in public settings. Illustrating this in relation to two unacquainted pedestrians passing each other on a footpath, Goffman notes that: "After a quick but open glance at a proper distance, the participants' looks are lowered for each other, and raised again only at the moment of passing . . . they should neither signal 'recognition', promising an openness for contact, nor should they be full of distrust and hatred" (Goffman 1963, p. 84). Hirschauer refers to this as a display of disinterestedness without regard (Hirschauer, 2005). This typically happens in a wide range of public settings where we move among strangers, such as on sidewalks in elevators or while lining up to make a purchase (Patterson & Webb, 2002).

Civil inattention (or polite ignoring) would sit at one end of the potential continuum of what can occur when strangers encounter each other in public settings. By contract, when strangers do interact with each other (nonverbally or verbally), what are the antecedents for this? A "baby in a pram" is one such catalyst, often observed to invoke a smile, verbal comment, or conversation between strangers. But companion animals seem to provide a similar trigger, and in the context of public settings such as sidewalks and parks, a dog being walked is a frequent catalyst for social interaction (Eddy, Hart, & Boltz, 1988; Katcher & Beck, 1983; McNicholas & Collis, 2000; Messent, 1983).

The type of social contact and interaction that might be facilitated or occur as a by-product of dog walking can be considered along a passive to proactive continuum (see Figure 4.2).

Figure 4.2. Continuum of social interaction potentially facilitated through dog walking.

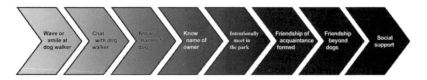

The nonverbal end of the spectrum includes gestures such as a nod, wave, smile, or other subtle forms of acknowledgement of another person. In a survey of residents (n=350: 56% dog owners, 44% non-dog owners) in a cluster of Perth (Western Australia) suburbs (Wood et al., 2008), dog owners (n=196: 56% dog owners) were more likely to report "waving to other people" at the park (73.9% of dog owners compared with 58.1% of non-dog owners). Dog owners were also slightly less likely to indicate that they felt they were being ignored by other people when at parks, compared with non-dog owners (75.2% and 78.4%, respectively). The social dividends of dog walking are not of course limited to humans, as emerged in focus groups undertaken in the United Kingdom, which found that many dog walkers choose to walk where they can anticipate meeting other dog walkers because they believe their dog enjoys socializing with other dogs (Edwards & Knight, 2006). Participants in the same study also noted that such environments provide social opportunities to meet others and converse themselves (Edwards & Knight, 2006). For example, dog walkers often only know each other by their dog (e.g., she's Max's owner or he's Bella's owner), and this illustrates the reciprocal relationship between the social interaction of dogs and dog walkers (Westgarth et al., 2010).

Moving along the social interaction continuum, the anecdotal stories of many dog owners are verified by research on dogs as a conversation trigger between strangers or casual acquaintances (Edwards & Knight, 2006; Messent, 1983; Robins, Sanders, & Cahill, 1991; Rogers, Hart, & Boltz, 1993). Several studies with an experimental design have been undertaken to compare social encounters experienced by people walking alone or with a dog, finding that those walking with a dog are far more likely to experience social contact and conversation with strangers than solitary walkers (McNicholas & Collis, 2000; Messent, 1983). Another study examined the behavior of pedestrians (n=1,800) when approaching a female experimenter who was sometimes alone and sometimes in the company of a dog (Labrador retriever pup, Labrador adult, rottweiler adult) (Wells, 2004). It was observed that the experimenter was more likely to be ignored whenever she was alone, compared with times in which she was walking one of the dogs.

The hypothesis that dogs are a disinhibitor for social exchange was also tested in a study that examined whether people in wheelchairs received more frequent social acknowledgement from able-bodied strangers if they were accompanied by a service dog (Hart & Hart, 1987). The authors found that both smiles and conversations from people passing by increased when a dog was present with the person in a wheelchair, concluding that service dogs reduced the tendency for able-bodied people to ignore or avoid people with disabilities (Hart & Hart, 1987). In another experimental study, respondents (n=45) were asked to view different images of an outdoor scene, only one of which depicted a person walking a dog, and asked to rate the pictures on several criteria. Respondents were more likely to indicate that the person in the pictures appeared happiest and most relaxed when depicted with a dog (Rossbach & Wilson, 1992). Such observational studies suggest that the presence of a dog appears to diminish some of the apprehension that people may inherently hold about "strangers." In an interview-based study (n=295) by Glasier (2009), respondents indicated that they were more likely to talk to a stranger with a dog than one without and that they trusted strangers more when they had a dog.

There is some empirical survey data corroborating the social lubrication provided by dogs (Lockwood, 1983; Messent, 1983). In the Perth social capital study (n=339), 50% of dog owners reported getting to know people as a result of their dog, and 84% talked to other pet owners when walking their dog (Wood et al., 2005). Furthermore, dog owners were significantly more likely to report having conversations with others when at a park compared with non-dog-owners (84.5% and 65.2%, respectively) (Wood et al., 2008). In a survey of dog walkers (n=120) visiting six parks in Victoria (Australia), 70% of respondents reported that they would always or mostly talk to other people when at the park, with the dog precipitating the conversation in most instances (94.2%) (Jackson, Mannix, Faga, & McDonald, 2005). In a recent U.S. study (Lee, Shepley, & Huang, 2009) almost 77% of respondents "strongly agreed" or "agreed" that a dog park provides opportunities to meet neighbors and build a sense of community by socializing with others. In this study, 26% of those surveyed identified socializing/talking as one of their main park activities when they are with a dog, second only to walking around the park (30%). These results were corroborated in an observational study of dog park participants in the same study (Lee et al., 2009).

Ethnographic research yields some deeper insight into the process and nature of interactions that take place between dog walkers. For example, Robins (Robins et al., 1991) documents his own experience as a participant (dog owner and walker) and observer at a local park over a three month period, and although the study is small in terms of the number of dog walkers observed (approximately 15 dog owners were observed consistently), the insights are nonetheless rich. Robins observed that it was the regular dog walkers who initiated conversations with newcomers to the park, and noted that such conversations initially focused on dog-related topics until the newcomer was welcomed as a "regular." Once accepted as a "regular," an expectation to be at the park when the "regulars" walked their dogs evolved, and Robins found that he was greeted upon arrival and leaving and any absence was noted (Robins et al., 1991).

So why is it that dogs appear to reduce inhibitions regarding social contact between strangers? One rationale proposed by Newby is that, "the presence of a pet seems to 'normalize' social situations, getting everyone through the ice-breaker stage to the point where they can risk directly engaging with the unfamiliar person" (Newby, 1997). Dogs are a practical "ice-breaker" providing people with a safe and neutral conversation starter (McNicholas & Collis, 2000). Another suggestion is that a person's perceived likability may be enhanced by the presence of a dog (Rossbach & Wilson, 1992). This resonates with the psychological concept of "attribution effect" or "fundamental attribution error" (Burger, 1991); the tendency to explain and value behavior (for example, dog walking) based on dispositional or personality-based traits or motives (for example, if liking or being liked by animals is seen culturally as a positive thing, then positive attributes are assigned to those observed with animals).

Companion animals are also a great leveler, transcending racial, cultural, geographic, age, and socioeconomic boundaries in terms of their ownership and impact (Wood et al., 2005). This is evident in the exchanges between dog owners of diverse backgrounds at a local park (Wood, 2009). The ability of dogs to precipitate conversation between neighbors or relative strangers is not merely a polite social nicety—such interactions can help to break down barriers and stereotypes about "others" and can play an important role in building trust and sense of community at the neighborhood level (Wood, 2010). As noted by one dog owner, "All status goes out the window. Dogs are an instant way to bond with someone without all the trappings of social mores" (Focus group participant [Wood, 2009]).

Looking beyond the perspective of the dog owner, Australian research also suggests that even people who do not own a dog themselves may view dogs as a social ice-breaker (Wood, Giles-Corti, Bulsara, & Bosch, 2007). Examples of dogs acting as social ice-breakers for non-pet owners include meeting or talking to a neighbor with a dog, chatting to dog owners at a local park, or talking to a dog walker who walks past the house:

> I like to see them as they come past walking their dogs. . . . there is always somebody out walking the dog and if you're out they always speak to you. (Focus Group participant [Wood et al., 2007])

> People walk through there all the time with their dogs and I get to know them. I've probably meet hundreds of people who go through there who speak to me every morning and every evening and I've made some quite good friends amongst some on the street. (Focus Group participant [Wood et al., 2007])

A recently published Japanese study also suggests that even having owned a dog in the past can have a long-term effect on social connectedness, with the authors finding that childhood experiences of dog ownership were positively related to sociality and enhanced companionship with others among elderly men in the study (Nagasawa & Ohta, 2010).

Friendship formation derived from dog walking facilitated interactions

Further along the social interaction continuum, social contact between humans instigated by a dog can facilitate the establishment of trust between people who are newly acquainted (Robins et al., 1991) and can precipitate people getting to know each other and forming friendships. In focus groups undertaken by Cutt as part of the DAPA study, many dog owners mentioned that walking with a dog was an excellent way to meet people and to get to know neighbors (Cutt, Giles-Corti, Knuiman, et al., 2008). For some, social interaction precipitated by dog walking led to long-term friendships (Cutt, Giles-Corti, Knuiman, et al., 2008). Making friends and meeting other dog walkers were also among benefits of dog walking cited by dog owners participating in qualitative research in the United Kingdom (Edwards & Knight, 2006). As noted by one dog walker, "When I moved to Perth I knew no-one and lost the support network I had built up in Melbourne. Thank goodness for the dogs, they were my ice-breakers and gave me a bond with total strangers who I soon called my friends" (Wood, 2009).

To date, there has been limited empirical research investigating friendships facilitated through dog walking. In one Australian survey of dog walkers (n=120) over one-third of respondents indicated they had got to know other dog owners as more than just a social acquaintance through walking their dog in a park, and some had formed friendships in which people met up with each other in a non-dog walking context (e.g., meeting up for dinner or for coffee) (Jackson et al., 2005). Comparing the experiences of people with and without dogs in the Western Australian PARKS study, 37.9% of dog owners indicated that they had made friends while at a park, compared with 26.5% of non-dog owners (Wood et al., 2008). In the Perth social capital study, pet owners were more likely than non-pet owners to "rarely or never" find it hard to get to know people (74.5% compared with 62.6%, respectively), and nearly 90% of pet owners indicated that they had gotten to know people in their suburb that they did not previously know. In the same study, the odds of more frequently feeling lonely were twice as high among non-pet owners compared with pet owners (Wood et al., 2005). While not yet researched, the growing number of social networking Web sites being used to connect dog owners both locally and internationally suggests that pets may also play a role in facilitating connectedness via the cyber realm.

Social support derived from dog walking facilitated interactions

At the "deeper" end of the social interaction continuum lies the concept of social support. There is a growing body of evidence linking both mental and physical health and well-being to social connectedness, social networks, and social support (Berkman, 1984; Berkman & Glass, 2000; Berkman, Glass, Brissette, & Seeman, 2000; Kawachi & Berkman, 2001; Lynch, 1977; Lynch, 2000; Tomaka, Thompson, & Palacios, 2006). Social support is one of ten key social determinants of health identified by the World Health Organization (Marmot & Wilkinson, 2006). Conversely, social isolation and loneliness can negatively affect health (Locher et al., 2005; Tomaka et al., 2006) and are risk factors for poor mental health. Social isolation and a lack of social support have also been linked to increased risk of cardiovascular heart disease, independent of other more established risk factors such as smoking and hypertension (Bunker et al., 2003).

The link between social support and health precedes its "discovery" in formal research studies, for as noted by Sartorius:

> Since the dawn of time, the survival of human beings has depended on the level of their integration into one or more mutually helpful communities.

> Those with social support and links with others live better than those
> who remain isolated. (Satorius, 2003)

Social support is often defined fairly loosely and measured as a composite, but this can mask the fact that social support often takes a number of different forms (Israel & McLeroy, 1985). A useful typology of social support is provided by House (1981), who identifies four main types:

Figure 4.3. Types of social support.

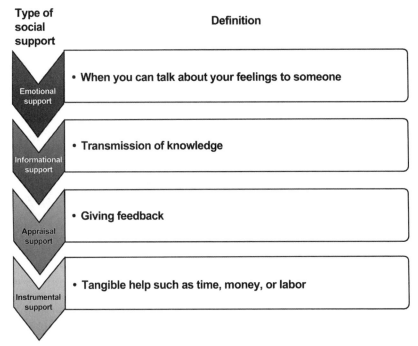

*Adapted from House, 1981; Israel & McLeroy, 1985.

Although the role of dogs and pets themselves in providing social support to their owners has been canvassed in the research to date, the concept has been far less considered in relation to whether dogs as a "third party" can facilitate networks of support among people. Anecdotal evidence suggests, however, that this can be the case, as exemplified in the following quotes:

> I came to Perth not knowing anyone. Luckily, I chose a suburb very
> close to the dog park where I met a very interesting, friendly and eclectic
> bunch of dog owners that saved my sanity. . . . Some days I thought I
> would die of loneliness and boredom and the only thing that would get
> me through was knowing that from 4-5 I could go to the park and talk

to real adults that had an interest in me as a person and that interest had started because of our mutual love of dogs." (Wood, 2009)

I am currently experiencing a family crisis. I have been offered help to look after my dog, legal advice, medical advice and advice from people who have experienced a similar situation. The dog mafia is extensive. I suspect the foregoing has certainly kept me sane!" (Wood, 2009)

Other anecdotes from dog owners suggest that the social contacts and networks forged through a dog park need not translate into friendships per se to be a source of social support, as reflected in the following quote from a focus group participant in the DAPA study:

> There is a lady that lives by herself and one night there was a thunderstorm and her electricity cut off and one of the walkers came to us and said "Can you help this lady?" We only knew her from the dog park. She was very frail and we just helped her out. But if she didn't come to the park no one would have known she was in trouble and she didn't have anyone else. . . . So people sort of watch out for each other and everyone knows each other. You can't really replace that. I mean you wouldn't have that if you didn't have the ability to walk your dog. (DAPA study focus group participant [Cutt, 2007])

Unfortunately there has been very little empirical research relating to social support derived from people meeting through dog walking, and the evidence that exists is mixed and only compares pet owners and non-pet owners rather than dog walkers and non-dog walkers. In the Perth social capital study, pet owners were more likely to "strongly agree" or "agree" with a statement pertaining to the general willingness of people to help each other out (85.0% of pet owners compared with 79.1% of non-pet owners), although this result did not reach statistical significance in multivariate analysis (Wood et al., 2005). Pet owners were also more likely to exchange favors with neighbors and were significantly less likely to report finding it hard to get to know people generally, compared with non-pet owners (Wood et al., 2005). However, in a United Kingdom study comparing dog and cat owners and non-pet owners, Collis et al. found that pet ownership did not significantly affect the size or composition of participants' social networks, concluding that casual interactions facilitated by dogs do not necessarily enhance social networks or social support (Collis, McNicholas, & Harker, 2003). The sample size for this study, however, was relatively small (52 dog owners, 44 cat owners, and 43 non-owners).

Further investigation (both qualitative and quantitative research) of the extent to which relationships forged through dogs and/or dog walking translates into actual social support is warranted. In particular, it would be useful for measures of social support to distinguish between different types of support (House, 1981), as it is plausible that exchanges of informational support (e.g., recommending a babysitter, dog sitter, or tradesperson) may occur more readily among people who are less well acquainted than deeper level emotional support (e.g., listening to or helping with personal problems). Although it is pertinent to note that in the qualitative dog walking quotes included above, all four types of social support are detectable.

Visible community presence and dog walking

The presence (or relative absence) of people "out and about" in neighborhoods, towns, and city streets conveys something about the social vitality of a place and its sense of community (Wallsjapser, 2007). The visible presence of people can also enhance both the actual and perceived safety of a community as embodied in the notion of "eyes on the street." As Jane Jacobs (1961) astutely observed, a well used city street is apt to be far safer than a deserted one, advocating that such public streets should have "eyes on them as continuously as possible." Referring to city streets, she noted, "A person must feel personally safe and secure among all these strangers . . . as if people fear them [the streets], they will use them less, which makes the streets still more unsafe" (Jacobs, 1961). Herein lies the paradox; if more people are out and about ("eyes on the street"), perceptions and actual safety may be enhanced, thereby encouraging more people to step beyond their front doors and into and around their neighborhood. Conversely, seeing few or no people out and about fuels concerns about the safety of the neighborhood and may further deter social interaction with community members and the opportunity to strengthen community ties.

Seeing people out walking their dogs, and the impetus dogs provide for people to be out walking in their streets and neighborhoods, can thus contribute to "eyes on the street" and in turn increase feelings of collective safety. As evident in the fear of crime literature, perceptions of crime and safety and fearfulness are influenced by many things, irrespective of actual crime rates or experiences (Hale, 1996; Wilson-Doenges, 2000). Moreover, fear of crime and not feeling safe can sometimes be as detrimental in a community as actual crime; if people are fearful they may be less likely to go out of their home or use local facilities, be reluctant to walk to destinations, or hesitant to interact with strangers or people they meet "in the street," particularly at night. Moreover, the more people "out walking," the safer the neighborhood is for those who walk (Wood & Giles-Corti, 2008). In the Perth social capital study, the visible presence of people "out and about," including dog walking, emerged as a positive marker of community safety. Conversely, deserted streets and parks conveyed negative impressions about safety, crime, and general sense of community (Wood et al., 2007). Importantly, a spillover effect is present, with community "out and aboutness" and its influence on perceptions of safety benefiting those both with and without dogs. As articulated by study participants:

> If you don't see anyone walking around the street or walking their dog or anything or only occasionally you see someone walking their dog down the street . . . it's like what is going on here? (Focus group participant [Wood et al., 2007])

> I think it would be very beneficial if we had more people on the street. While there is a downside as far as enforcement, there are upsides in regard to neighborhood watch. People being out on the streets, crime prevention, communities coming together and being exposed to each other, neighbors talking, dogs bring down barriers. It's the same as being a mother with kids at school. (DAPA study, in-depth interviews [Cutt, 2007])

In the DAPA study focus groups, some participants talked about feeling safer when walking with their dog and suggested dog ownership may be a deterrent for local crime (Cutt, Giles-Corti, & Knuiman, 2008). Edwards and Knight found that the majority of focus group participants indicated feeling safer having their dogs with them, with female participants in particular expressing concerns about walking alone or in the dark (Edwards & Knight, 2006). In terms of empirical data, in the Perth social capital study, 63.6% of dog owners indicated that owning a dog helped them to feel safer when out walking (Wood et al., 2007), while in a U.S. study, women were three times more likely to walk for exercise or walk a dog in the neighborhood if neighborhood safety was average as opposed to below average (Suminski, Poston, Petosa, Stevens, & Katzenmoyer, 2005).

There is growing research and intervention interest in the capacity of dogs to encourage more walking by owners and increased use of parks and open spaces for physical activity (Bauman, Schroeder, Furber, & Dobson, 2001; Thorpe et al., 2006; Cutt, 2007 #4866; Christian (née Cutt) et al., 2010). While less considered to date, it is also plausible that the visible presence of dogs being walked, the accompanying social exchanges, and the impetus dogs provide for people to be out walking in the streets and parks, contributes to increased feelings of collective safety and perceptions of sense of community (Wood et al., 2005). This draws attention to the accumulated community benefits that can arise from dog walking, over and above the individual benefits to dogs and their owners. Thus, these "spillover" effects of dog ownership and dog walking on the broader community warrant further research attention.

Civic engagement, community involvement, and dog walking

It is often lamented that community involvement and volunteering are on the decline in many countries, with busyness, individualism, and a loss of sense of community commonly cited culprits. The negative repercussions of such trends for the social fabric of society were brought into the public spotlight in Robert Putnam's book entitled *Bowling Alone: The Collapse and Revival of American Community*, fuelling a renaissance of interest in the notion of civil society (Cox, 1995; Putnam, 1996). Civic engagement is one of the markers of a civil society and relates to the capacity of individuals to be concerned and active within the community, which in turn creates the "capital" from which others can benefit. While active citizens contribute to the community by the "good things that they do" (e.g., volunteering), civic engagement also contributes to the building of trust and networks. In the Perth study (Wood et al., 2005), survey respondents were asked whether they had taken action on a local issue(s), such as attending a local action meeting, writing to a newspaper or politician about a local issue, or signing a petition. Pet owners were 57% more likely to be engaged than non-pet owners on this civic engagement scale (Wood et al., 2005). It might be surmised that dog owners may have an active interest and involvement in aspects of community that directly impact on them, such as access to parks and open space for walking dogs or regulations about dog ownership. However, in this study, the civic engagement scale was not specific to community-based dog walking issues and actions (Wood et al., 2005).

Nonetheless, many of the issues that provoke the concern and interest of dog walkers inevitably are of benefit to the community more broadly. Dog walkers have a vested interest, for example, in the availability and maintenance of local parks and open space, adding their "voice" to the broader imperative for access to parks, open space, and opportunities to come into contact with nature. This can also translate into volunteering. For example, one local government in Western Australia runs an "Adopt-A-Park" program that aims to promote community ownership, pride, and safety for its local parks and reserves (City of Stirling, 2009); a high proportion of the supporters signed up to this program have a dog and attend parks regularly with their dog. Activities undertaken by "Adopt-A-Park" supporters include picking up litter, removing or reporting graffiti or damaged equipment, and providing a positive presence in parks (City of Stirling, 2009).

In addition to more formalized volunteering through programs such as "Adopt-A-Park," the social fabric of a community is also reflected in the extent to which people informally and incidentally look out for each other and for the community. This may often go unseen, but nonetheless be of broader community benefit, as illustrated by the quotes from some focus group participants in the Perth study:

> We used to go at night to the park with the dog . . . to pick up syringes that have been used. And if they hadn't been picked up they probably would have been there the next morning. (Wood et al., 2007)

> It was originally Neighborhood Watch, but now it's just an old man with a big dog that keeps a big note pad and runs around checking on everyone. (Wood et al., 2007)

Interviews with local government employees in the DAPA study also illustrate the role dog owners play in upholding and self-regulating responsible dog ownership in parks and open space areas, as reflected in the following quote from a participating ranger:

> It's worked out really well because they (dog owners) do a lot for us if we aren't there, because you can't be there 24 hours a day. If they see somebody not picking up after their dog they will go and tell them straight off and quite a lot of the women actually do pick up after other people that they don't physically see or catch and I give them extra bags when I am down there and incentives. (Cutt, Giles-Corti, Knuiman, & Adams, 2006, p. 8)

Healthy social urban design and dog walking

There is growing recognition of the role of the built environment in health and social well-being. The built environment can help to shape the social dimension of a community with poorly built environments having a corrosive effect on social fabric. Urban planning paradigms such as "New Urbanism" place a strong emphasis on creating pedestrian-friendly neighborhoods and fostering sense of community (Joongsub & Kaplan, 2004; Lund, 2003). Recent reports such as the U.S. Transportation Research Board's report on the built environment and physical activity (TRB, 2005) and "The State of Australian Cities" (Infrastructure Australia Major Cities Unit, 2010) emphasize the importance of livability and quality of life in the planning of cities, and urban planners, developers, and local government are increasingly requesting evidence-based guidance on designing health-enhancing communities.

Healthy social urban design is also important for dog walking. As articulated by Wallsjasper (author of *The Great Neighborhood Book*), "When you create a neighborhood that's friendly to dogs, it's friendly to people, too. The traffic is not speeding and dangerous. There are green places to hang out and walk. So dogs are a good indicator species" (Hage, 2007).

Findings from the DAPA study suggest that dog owners are attracted to attributes of suburbs and parks that are equally valued by everyone: walkable streets and parks that are attractive, well lit, safe, and close to home (Cutt, Giles-Corti, Wood, Knuiman, & Burke, 2008). Conversely, features of the physical environment that support physical activity and walking in the population generally (such as park attractiveness, size, accessibility, and safety) (Giles-Corti & Donovan, 2003; Owen, Humpel, Leslie, Bauman, & Sallis, 2004) are also important for dog walkers (Cutt et al., 2007; Lee et al., 2009).

Demand for more walkable and green communities is not only being driven by those in public health, but also by sectors concerned with environmental sustainability and the adverse environmental and social problems associated with traffic congestion, pollution, and urban sprawl (Duany, Plater-Zyberk, & Speck, 2000). A walkable community is one that has well-connected streets, high density residential housing, and a mix of land uses (e.g., shops and green spaces) (Giles-Corti, Timperio, Bull, & Pikora, 2005; Owen et al., 2007). A walkable community is also important for sense of community and may provide a more supportive physical and social environment to encourage dog owners to walk with their dog and interact with other owners and nonowners. As noted by Nozzi, "The serendipitous experience of bumping into those who live on your street frequently occurs when one walks, but nearly vanishes when one drives a car. Healthy neighborliness is a necessary ingredient if sense of community is to be achieved" (Nozzi, 2007, p. 1). Dog walkers may be one of the important ingredients in healthy neighborliness that facilitates sense of community and social capital. Whether watching the beloved family dog run freely at a park or simply being surrounded by nature, taking the dog for a walk to the local park or in natural settings also satisfies an innate human desire to connect with nature and living things (Cutt et al., 2007). The human need for an intimate bond with nature and the natural world is often referred to as the biophilia theory (Katcher & Wilkins, 1993). A restorative space such as the local park provides dog owners with the opportunity to connect with living things (e.g., their dog and the natural environment) (Cutt et al., 2007).

Future research

With growing recognition of the importance of the social and community environment for health and quality of life, greater research momentum around the role of dogs and dog walking in facilitating social interaction and contributing to the social fabric of communities is warranted. Attention to research rigor is also warranted, as in many areas of human-animal interaction research, the generalizability of existing research is often hindered by methodological limitations such as small sample sizes.

As postulated by McNicholas et al. (2005), in considering the health benefits of companion animals, a broader definition of health is required, one that looks beyond merely physical health outcomes, to encompass the broader role of pets in people's lives, including dimensions of well-being (physical and mental) and a sense of social integration. From a research perspective, questions relating to social contact that might arise during dog walking could be readily included in future studies investigating dog walking as a form of human and canine physical activity. Similarly, surveys of community social capital and sense of community are not uncommon, and represent an opportunity to include questions about companion animals (e.g., dog ownership, social interactions facilitated by dog walking).

Along with the merits of further research and intervention interest in the role of dogs and other companion animals as social catalysts, it is also timely to expand our view of the way in which dog walking might enhance mental health. In companion animal research to date, the mental health benefits have primarily focused on those arising directly from owning or having contact with animals (e.g., reduced loneliness, companionship, social support, and consolation in times of bereavement). Given the mounting evidence associating social networks, social support, sense of community, and reduced isolation with better mental health generally, the role of dog walking as a conduit for some of this warrants more rigorous investigation. Importantly, this need not be confined to "animal-specific" studies, but could entail the incorporation of dog-related questions into broader community and population surveys relating to mental health determinants or community well-being.

Conclusion

While there is an accumulating body of research around the benefits of dog walking to both dogs and their owners, there is also emerging evidence of a link to the social fabric of society. This includes the role of dog walking in facilitating social interactions, social support, and sense of community, benefitting not only dog walkers themselves, but having a ripple effect into the broader community. From an intervention perspective, there are clear synergies between interventions promoting dog walking as a conduit for human (and canine) physical activity, and the potential role of dogs as facilitators of social and community interaction. More broadly, planning and designing for walkable, green, and socially vibrant communities will benefit dog and non-dog owners alike. In summary: Dogs, then, can provide more companionship for humans than merely their own company. They are also an antidote for the human anonymity of the public places of our contemporary society.

Acknowledgments

Both authors are currently supported by a National Health and Medical Research Council (Australia) capacity building grant (#458668).The research assistance of Katharine I'Anson and Penny Ivery in the preparation of this chapter is gratefully acknowledged.

References

Albery, N. (2001). *The world's greatest ideas: An encyclopedia of social inventions.* Gabriola Island, BC, Canada: New Society Publishers.

Bauman, A., Schroeder, J., Furber, S., & Dobson, A. (2001). The epidemiology of dog walking: An unmet need for human and canine health. *Medical Journal of Australia, 175,* 632-634.

Beck, A. M., & Katcher, A. H. (2003). Future directions in human–animal bond research. *American Behavioral Scientist, 47*(1), 79-93.

Berkman, L. (1984). Assessing the physical health effects of social networks and social support. *Ann Rev Public Health, 5,* 413-432.

Berkman, L., & Glass, T. (2000). Social integration, social networks, social support, and health. In L. Berkman & I. Kawachi (Eds.), *Social epidemiology.* New York: Oxford University Press.

Berkman, L. F., Glass, T., Brissette, I., & Seeman, T. E. (2000). From social integration to health: Durkheim in the new millennium. *Social Science & Medicine, 51*(6), 843-857.

Bunker, S., Colquhoun, D., Esler, M., Hickie, I., Hunt, D., Jelinek, V., et al. (2003). "Stress" and coronary heart disease: Psychosocial risk factors. *Medical Journal of Australia, 178*(17 March), 272-276.

Burger, J. M. (1991). Changes in attributions over time: The ephemeral fundamental attribution error. *Social Cognition, 9*(2), 182-193.

Christian (née Cutt), H., Giles-Corti, B., & Knuiman, M. (2010). "I'm just a'-walking the dog" correlates of regular dog walking. *Family and Community Health, 33*(1), 44-52.

City of Stirling. (2009). Adopt-A-Park. Retrieved from http://www.stirling.wa.gov.au/home/services/Volunteers+at+Stirling/Adopt-A-Park.htm

Collis, G., McNicholas, J., & Harker, R. (2003). Could enhanced social networks explain the association between pet ownership and health? *Unpublished paper,* Department of Psychology, University of Warwick.

Cox, E. (1995). *A truly civil society: 1995 Boyer lectures.* Sydney: Australian Broadcasting Corporation.

Cutt, H. (2007). *The relationship between dog ownership and physical activity.* Doctor of Philosophy, University of Western Australia, Perth.

Cutt, H., Giles-Corti, B., & Knuiman, M. (2008). Encouraging physical activity through dog walking: Why don't some owners walk with their dog? *Preventive Medicine, 46*(2), 120-126.

Cutt, H., Giles-Corti, B., Knuiman, M., & Adams, T. (2006). Who's taking who for a walk? Dog walking and regulation in West Australian loval government. Paper presented at the 18th National Urban Animal Management Conference, Hobart, Tasmania.

Cutt, H., Giles-Corti, B., Knuiman, M., & Burke, V. (2007). Dog ownership, health and physical activity: A critical review of the literature. *Health Place, 13*(1), 261-272

Cutt, H., Giles-Corti, B., Knuiman, M., & Pikora, T. (2008). Physical activity behaviour of dog owners: Development and reliability of the dogs and physical activity (DAPA) tool. *Journal of Physical Activity & Health, 5*(Supp 1), S83-S89.

Cutt, H., Knuiman, M., & Giles-Corti, B. (2008). Does getting a dog increase recreational walking? *International Journal of Behavioral Nutrition and Physical Activity, 5*(1), 17.

Cutt, H. E., Giles-Corti, B., Wood, L. J., Knuiman, M. W., & Burke, V. (2008). Barriers and motivators for owners walking their dog: Results from qualitative research. *Health Promotion Journal of Australia, 19*(2), 118-124.

Duany, A., Plater-Zyberk, E., & Speck, J. (2000). *Suburban nation: The rise of sprawl and the decline of the American dream.* New York: North Point Press.

Eddy, J., Hart, L. A., & Boltz, R. P. (1988). The effects of service dogs on social acknowledgments of people in wheelchairs. *Journal of Psychology, 122*(1), 39-45.

Edwards, V., & Knight, S. (2006). Understanding the psychology of walkers with dogs: New approaches to better management. Hampshire: University of Portsmouth.

Giles-Corti, B., & Donovan, R. J. (2003). The relative influence of individual, social environmental and physical environmental correlates of walking. *American Journal of Public Health, 93*, 1183-1189.

Giles-Corti, B., Timperio, A., Bull, F., & Pikora, T. (2005). Understanding physical activity environmental correlates: Increased specificity for ecological models. *Exercise and Sport Sciences Reviews, 33*(4), 175-181.

Glasier, A. (2009). Canine catalysts: Public perceptions of four dog breeds and the ability of dogs to act as a social bridge between strangers. Paper presented at the ISAZ Podium Presentation.

Goffman, E. (1963). *Behavior in public places: Notes on the social organization of gatherings.* New York: Free Press.

Hage, D. (2007). A simple path to strong neighborhoods. *Star Tribune.* Retrieved November 2007, from http://www.startribune.com/opinion/commentary/11764191.html

Hale, C. (1996). Fear of crime: A review of the literature. *International Review of Victimology, 4*, 79-150.

Hanifan, L. (1920). *The community centre.* Boston: Silver, Burdette and Co.

Hart, L., & Hart, B. L. (1987). Socializing effects of service dogs for people with disabilities. *Anthrozoos, 1*, 41-44.

Hirschauer, S. (2005). On doing being a stranger: The practical constitution of civil inattention. *Journal for the Theory of Social Behaviour, 35*(1), 41-67.

House, J. S. (1981). *Work stress and social support.* Reading, MA: Addison-Wesley Company.

Infrastructure Australia Major Cities Unit. (2010). State of Australian Cities 2010. Canberra: Commonwealth of Australia.

Israel, B. A., & McLeroy, K. R. (1985). Social networks and social support: Implications for health-education-introduction. [Editorial material]. *Health Education Quarterly, 12*(1), 1-4.

Jackson, D., Mannix, J., Faga, P., & McDonald, G. (2005). Overweight and obese children: Mothers' strategies. *Journal of Advanced Nursing, 52*(1), 6-13.

Jacobs, J. (1961). *The death and life of the great American cities.* New York: Random House.

Joongsub, K., & Kaplan, R. (2004). Physical and psychological factors in sense of community: New urbanist Kentlands and nearly Orchard Village. *Environment and Behaviour, 36*(3), 313-340.

Katcher, A., & Wilkins, G. G. (1993). Dialogue with animals: Its nature and culture. In S. R. Kellert & E. O. Wilson (Eds.), *The biophilia hypothesis* (pp. 173-200). Washington, DC: Island Press.

Katcher, A. H., & Beck, A. M. (1983). *New perspectives on our lives with companion animals*. Philadelphia: University of Pennsylvania Press.

Kawachi, I., & Berkman, L. F. (2001). Social ties and mental health. *Journal of Urban Health, 78*(3), 458 - 467.

Lee, H.-S., Shepley, M., & Huang, C.-S. (2009). Evaluation of off-leash dog parks in Texas and Florida: A study of use patterns, user satisfaction, and perception. *Landscape and Urban Planning, 92*(3-4), 314-324.

Locher, J., Ritchie, C., Roth, D., Sawyer Baker, P., Bodner, E., & Allman, R. (2005). Social isolation, support, and capital and nutritional risk in an older sample: Ethnic and gender differences. *Social Science and Medicine, 60*, 747-761.

Lockwood, R. (1983). The influence of animals on social perception. In A. H. Katcher & A. M. Beck (Eds.), *New perspectives on our lives with companion animals* (pp. 64-71). Philadelphia: University of Pennsylvania Press.

Lund, H. (2003). Testing the claims of new urbanism: Local access, pedestrian travel, and neighboring behaviors. *Journal of the American Planning Association, 69*(4), 414-429.

Lynch, J. J. (1977). *The broken heart: The medical consequences of loneliness*. New York: Basic Book.

Lynch, J. J. (2000). *A cry unheard: New insights into the medical consequences of loneliness*. Baltimore, MD: Bancroft Press.

Marmot, M., & Wilkinson, R. (2006). *Social determinants of health (Second Ed.)*. Oxford: Oxford University Press.

McNicholas, J., & Collis, G. M. (2000). Dogs as catalysts for social interactions: Robustness of the effect. *British Journal of Psychology, 91*(1), 61-70.

McNicholas, J., Gilbey, A., Rennie, A., Ahmedzai, S., Dono, J., & Ormerod, E. (2005). Pet ownership and human health: A brief review of evidence and issues. *BMJ, 331*, 252-255.

Messent, P. R. (1983). Social facilitation of contact with other people by pet dogs. In A. H. Katcher & A. M. Beck (Eds.), *New perspectives on our lives with companion animals* (pp. 37-46). Philadelphia: University of Pennsylvania Press.

Nagasawa, M., & Ohta, M. (2010). The influence of dog ownership in childhood on the sociality of elderly Japanese men. *Animal Science Journal, 81*(3), 377-383.

Newby, J. (1997). *The pact for survival: Humans and their companions*. Sydney: ABC Books.

Nozzi, D. (2007). Measuring walkable urbanity. Retrieved from http://www.walkablestreets.com/urbanity.htm

Owen, N., Cerin, E., Leslie, E., duToit, L., Coffee, N., Frank, L. D., et al. (2007). Neighborhood walkability and the walking behavior of Australian adults. *American Journal of Preventive Medicine, 33*(5), 387-395.

Owen, N., Humpel, N., Leslie, E., Bauman, A., & Sallis, J. (2004). Understanding environmental influences on walking: Review and research agenda. *American Journal of Preventive Medicine, 27*(1), 67-76.

Patterson, M. L., & Webb, A. (2002). Passing encounters: Patterns of recognition and avoidance in pedestrians. *Basic and applied social psychology, 24*(1), 57.

Podberscek, A. L. (2000). *The relationships between people and pets.* Cambridge: Cambridge University Press.

Putnam, R. (1996). The strange disappearance of civic America. *The American Prospect, 7,* 1-18.

Robins, D., Sanders, C., & Cahill, S. (1991). Dogs and their people: Pet-facilitated interaction in a public setting. *Journal of Contemporary Ethnography, 20*(1), 3-25.

Rogers, J., Hart, L. A., & Boltz, R. P. (1993). The role of pet dogs in casual conversations of elderly adults. *The Journal of Social Psychology, 133,* 265-277.

Rossbach, K. A., & Wilson, J. P. (1992). Does a dog's presence make a person appear more likeable? *Anthrozoos, 5*(1), 40-51.

Satorius, N. (2003). Social capital and mental health. *Current Opinion in Psychiatry, 16*(Suppl. 2), S101-S105.

Suminski, R. R., Poston, W. S. C., Petosa, R. L., Stevens, E., & Katzenmoyer, L. M. (2005). Features of the neighborhood environment and walking by US adults. *American Journal of Preventive Medicine, 28*(2), 149-155.

Thorpe, R. J., Kreisle, R. A., Glickman, L. T., Simonsick, E. M., Newman, A. B., & Kritchevsky, S. (2006). Physical activity and pet ownership in year 3 of the Health ABC Study. *Journal of Aging and Physical Activity, 14,* 154-168.

Thorpe, R. J., Simonsick, E. M., Brach, J. S., Ayonayon, H., Satterfield, S., Harris, T. B., et al. (2006). Dog ownership, walking behavior, and maintained mobility in late life. *Journal of the American Geriatrics Society, 54*(9), 1419-1424.

Tomaka, J., Thompson, S., & Palacios, R. (2006). The relation of social isolation, loneliness, and social support to disease outcomes among the elderly. *Journal of Aging and Health, 18,* 359.

TRB. (2005). *Does the built environment influence physical activity? Examining the evidence—special report 282.* Washington, DC: Transportation Research Board.

Walljasper, J. (2007). *The great neighborhood book.* Gabriola Island, BC, Canada: New Society.

Wells, D. L. (2004). The facilitation of social interactions by domestic dogs. *Anthrozoos, 17,* 340-352.

Westgarth, C., Christley, R. M., Pinchbeck, G. L., Gaskell, R. M., Dawson, S., & Bradshaw, J. W. S. (2010). Dog behaviour on walks and the effect of use of the leash. *Applied Animal Behaviour Science, 124*(1-2), 16-27.

Wilson-Doenges, G. (2000). An exploration of sense of community and fear of crime in gated communities. *Environment and Behaviour, 32*(5), 597-611.

Wise, A. (2008). "It's just an attitude that you feel": Inter-ethnic habitus before the Cronulla riots. In G. Noble (Ed.), *Lines in the sand: The Cronulla riots and the limits of Australian multiculturalism.* Sydney, Australia: Institute of Criminology Press.

Wood, L. (2006). *Social capital, mental health and the environments in which people live (PhD thesis).* The University of Western Australia, Perth.

Wood, L. (2010). Community benefits of human animal interactions . . . the ripple effect. In P. McCardle et al. (Eds.), *The role of pets in children's lives: Human-animal interaction in child development, health, and therapeutic intervention.* Baltimore, MD: Brookes Publishing.

Wood, L. (Ed.). (2009). *Living well together: How companion animals can help strengthen social fabric.* Melbourne: Petcare Information and Advisory Service and Centre for the Built Environment and Health, School of Population Health, The University of Western Australia.

Wood, L., & Giles-Corti, B. (2008). Is there a place for social capital in the psychology of health and place? *Journal of Environmental Psychology, 28*(2), 154-163.

Wood, L., Giles-Corti, B., & Bulsara, M. (2005). The pet connection: Pets as a conduit for social capital? *Social Science & Medicine, 61*(6), 1159-1173.

Wood, L., Walker, N., I'Anson, K., Ivery, P., French, S., & Giles-Corti, B. (2008). PARKS: Parks and reserves Kwinana study: The use and role of parks within the town of Kwinana. Centre for the Built Environment and Health, The University of Western Australia, Perth.

Wood, L. J., Giles-Corti, B., Bulsara, M. K., & Bosch, D. (2007). More than a furry companion: The ripple effect of companion animals on neighborhood interactions and sense of community. *Society and Animals, 15*(1), 43-56.

Chapter 5

Dog walking as physical activity for older adults

Roland J. Thorpe, Jr., Hayley E. Christian, and Adrian Bauman

Over the past two decades there has been an increasing interest in understanding the role of pets in the lives of older adults. There is a body of evidence suggesting that pets may improve psychological, social, and physical health of persons of all ages (Boldt & Dellmann-Jenkins, 1992). These health effects include conditions that have an increased prevalence among older adults (ages 65 and older) such as cardiovascular disease, dementia, and disability. Therefore, older adults might specifically benefit from companion animals (Berkman et al., 1986; Boldt & Dellmann-Jenkins, 1992; Branch & Jette, 1981; Estes, 1969; Jette & Branch, 1981; Murrell, Himmelfarb, & Wright, 1983). According to the Centers for Disease Control and Prevention's National Center for Health Statistics, more than 26 million Americans over 65 are not hospitalized or living in a nursing home, and about one-third of these people live alone (Siegel, 1993). Furthermore, 14% of individuals ages 65 and older in the U.S. own pets. This suggests that these pets may be an important component of their social support system. Thus, the population of adults 65 years of age and older should be a focus of research of the potential health implications of human-animal relations (Siegel, 1993). The purpose of the chapter is to delve into the literature examining the relationship among dog ownership, dog walking, and health in community-dwelling older adults (referred to hereafter as older adults).

There has been an abundance of anecdotal reports on the benefits of companion animals and human health, but there have been limited number of controlled scientific studies (Garrity, Stallones, Marx, & Johnson, 1989; Lago, Delaney, Miller, & Grill, 1989; Marx, Stallones, & Garrity, 1987; Ory

& Goldberg, 1983; Robb & Stegman, 1983; Rowan, 1991; Siegel, 1990) to explain this relationship. The results of these studies have been inconsistent in part due to a lack of controls, or inaccurate measurement of exposures and outcomes (Boldt & Dellmann-Jenkins, 1992; Katcher, 1982; Serpell, 1991). Another shortcoming in earlier work is the failure to specify a theoretical framework underlying research hypotheses for the association between pet ownership and health benefits (Garrity et al., 1989). As far back as 1987, the National Institutes of Health (NIH), in a report on *The Health Benefits of Pets*, stated that pet exposure should be considered as a possible protective factor in scientific studies of human health (NIH, 1988) and more importantly, that research is needed to test explanatory models for understanding health benefits of human-animal interaction (HAI) in older persons. More recently, in 2007, a group of investigators convened at the NIH to discuss the state of the HAI literature. In a recent book that reports on findings from this meeting, it was stated that pets are an important part of society and that an understanding of HAI should be a public health priority. Furthermore, there was a consensus among the investigators that a paradigm shift is needed to move beyond studies that merely examine correlates of pet ownership to longitudinal cohort studies and intervention studies. This is a necessary first step in HAI research in understanding the mechanism(s) that underlie the association between pet/dog ownership and improved human health. Hence explanatory models linking pets to health benefits are a key objective in HAI research. One suggested theory is that pet ownership substitutes for human social support and buffers stress, which in turn produces health benefits (Dembicki, 1995; Garrity et al., 1989; Siegel, 1990; Stallones, Marx, Garrity, & Johnson, 1990). An alternative hypothesis is that pets encourage behaviors that modify the development of age-related diseases, and thus preserves physical function. Moreover, the idea that pet ownership, specifically dog ownership, may provide health benefits in older adults by encouraging increased physical activity may be valid.

Thus, the aim of this chapter is to discuss the interrelationships among dog ownership, dog walking, and health indicators in older adults. Specifically, this chapter will be divided into three sections: 1) a brief overview of the health benefits of physical activity among older adults; 2) physical activity as a mechanism for the relationship between dog ownership and health benefits; and 3) future directions in enhancing our understanding of the relationship between dog walking and health in older adults.

Health benefits of physical activity among older adults

According to the first U.S. Surgeon's General report on physical activity and health, (U.S. Department of Health and Human Services, 1996) and the Healthy People 2010 report (U.S. Department of Health and Human Services, 2001), beneficial effects of physical activity are evident throughout life. Physical activity is defined as any voluntary body movement that burns calories (U.S. Department of Health and Human Services, 1999). It is an appealing lifestyle modification that is recommended by federal agencies for people of all ages to reduce the risk of dying prematurely, developing certain chronic conditions such as high blood pressure, type 2 diabetes, and improving overall well-being (Chobanian et al., 2003; U.S. Department of Health and Human Services, 1996; U.S. Department of Health and Human Services, 2001). The link between physical activity and health has been established in epidemiologic studies (Berlin & Colditz, 1990; Powell, Thompson, Caspersen, & Kendrick, 1987). Moreover, recent studies have shown participation in leisure activities unrelated to fitness increases survival and has other promising health benefits such as less disability among socially engaged older adults (Koenig, Hays, & Larson, 1999; Mendes de Leon, Glass, & Berkman, 2003; Musick, Herzog, & House, 1999). According to the Surgeon General Report on Physical Activity and Health (1996), older adults can achieve many health benefits through a minimum of 30 minutes of activity for five or more days (preferably daily). They can also benefit from strength training activities by preventing or reducing the number of falls, maintaining or building balance, strength, or flexibility, all of which are essential to maintenance of performing tasks in daily life. Popular forms of low levels of physical activity among older adults include walking with or without a pet, gardening, and yard work (U.S. Department of Health and Human Services, 1996). The health benefits that can be achieved from this moderate amount of physical activity vary from an increase in bone mineral density (Gregg, Pereira, & Caspersen, 2000), a decrease in low density lipoprotein (LDL) (U.S. Department of Health and Human Services, 2001), lower blood pressure (Mensink, Ziese, & Kok, 1999; Rauramaa et al., 1995; Tanaka, Reiling, & Seals, 1998; U.S. Department of Health and Human Services, 1996; U.S. Department of Health and Human Services, 2001), a decrease in dementia (Weih et al., 2009), preventing falls (Heesch, Byles, & Brown, 2008; Laforest et al., 2009), an increase in high density lipoprotein (HDL) (Houde & Melilo, 2002), improved cognitive function (Gillum & Obisesan, 2010; Lautenschlager et al., 2008; Williamson et al., 2009), general well-being (U.S. Department of Health and Human Services, 1996), reduction in cardiovascular-related mortality (Andersen, Schnohr, Schroll, & Hein, 2000; Ferrucci et al., 1999; Hakim et al., 1998), and preservation of mobility and physical capacity (Clark, 1996; Simonsick et al., 1993). With successful promotion among individuals and within communities, physical activity can be an effective intervention for treating and preventing chronic conditions and maintaining functional capacity because it is cost-effective and there are very few, if any, adverse effects compared to drug therapy.

Health benefits of pet ownership among older adults

Currently, 64 million (62%) U.S. households have a pet including dogs (39%), cats (33%), freshwater fish (13%), birds (6%), small animals (5%), reptiles (4%), and saltwater fish (.7%) (American Pet Products Association, 2009). Among individuals 65 years of age and older in the U. S., it is estimated that 14% own a pet (American Pet Products Manufacturers Association, 2009). Dogs and cats are popular pets among older adults in the U.S. (American Pet Products Association, 2009). However the prevalence of pet ownership in studies examining only older adults varied from 23% to 53% (Table 5.1). The variation in pet ownership prevalence among these studies appears to be inversely related to sample size. In other words, a larger prevalence of pet ownership is evident in the smaller and possibly more selected studies. Also, the prevalence of pet ownership varies because pet ownership may be related to the underlying health of older adults—that is, declining health with age may discourage pet ownership. Regardless, given the proportion (14%) of older adults in the U.S. who own a pet, even a small positive influence of pet ownership on human health could have public health significance. Furthermore, the U.S. population 65 years of age and older is increasing with the most notable segment being those of 85 years of age and older. Thus understanding how factors such as dog ownership and dog walking enhance longevity and independent living among community-dwelling older adults is likely to become increasingly important as the population ages.

Physical activity as a mechanism for the health benefits of dog ownership

There is a paucity of studies examining the relationship between physical activity and pet/dog ownership, and this number decreases even more when focusing only on older adults. Therefore, in this section we elected to describe all the studies examining pet/dog ownership and physical activity. Research has speculated that the link between pet ownership and improved health could be

Table 5.1. Selected characteristics of studies examining the relationship between pet ownership and health that contain older adults.

Author and Year	Population	Study Design	Age Range	Percent of Pet
Ory and Goldberg, 1983	1,073 women in Washington County, Maryland	CS	65-75 years old	36% (388 pet owners)
Robb and Stegman, 1983	56 veterans receiving home health services	CS	20-93 years old	46% (26 pet owners)
Lawton et al., 1984	3,996 seniors from the National Senior Citizen 1968	CS	65 years old and over	23% (959 pet owners)
Goldmeir, 1986	144 elderly women	CS	NA	52% (76 pet owners)
Garrity et al., 1989	1,232 households from a national probability sample	CS	65 years old and over	33% (408 pet owners)
Lago et al., 1989	355 rural, community-dwelling years	P	50-90	38% (136 pet owners)
Siegel, 1990	938 Medicare enrollees	P	65 years old and over	36% (345 pet owners)
Dembicki and Anderson, 1996	127 participants in north central Colorado	CS	60 years old and over	53% (44 pet owners)
Jorm et al., 1997	594 respondents dwelling in Australia.	CS	74-79 years old	28 % (169 pet owners)
Raina et al., 1999	1,054 community-dwelling Canadians	P	65 years old and over	27 % (286 pet owners)
Norris et al., 1999	532 individuals in predetermined Illinois zip code areas	CS	53-96 years old	22% (115 pet owners)

*CS=Cross-Sectional Study; P=Prospective Study; E=Experimental Study; NA=Not available.

due to increased physical activity. For example, in an Australian cross-sectional study of adults 20 to 60 years of age the authors suggested that a possible explanation for the lower systolic blood pressure, plasma cholesterol, and triglyceride levels in pet owners compared with non-pet owners was due to an increase in physical activity among pet owners compared with non-pet owners (Anderson, Reid, & Jennings, 1992). A separate study, using data from the Australian People and Pets Survey Headley (1999), examined the cross-sectional relationship between 606 pet owners (dogs or cats) and physician utilization and medication usage. In this cross-sectional study of 1,011 Australian residents ages 16 and over, the authors found that dog and cat owners, on average, make fewer annual visits to the doctor compared to non-pet owners and are less likely to be on medication when compared to non-pet owners. Also in this study, the authors noted that dog ownership could provide a further benefit to improved health because dog owners walked four times a week compared with 2.5 times for non-pet owners. Furthermore, in another Australian study of 894 adults 25 to 64 years old, dog owners (n=410) walked 18 minutes more per week than non-pet owners (n=484). These findings suggest that if all dog owners walked their dogs, there would be a substantial decrease in disease and an annual health care cost savings of 175 million dollars (Bauman, Russell, Furber, & Dobson, 2001). In 2006, Thorpe and colleagues established a link between dog ownership and physical activity in older adults. Specifically they found that dog owners had a greater frequency and longer duration of casual walks than non-pet and non-dog owners (Thorpe et al., 2006). They also noted the importance of testing physical activity as a mechanism for the association between dog ownership and physical activity among older adults. However, while results from each of these studies found both increased health benefits and physical activity among pet owners, none of them tested whether physical activity was an explanatory mechanism between pet ownership and health benefits.

Only one study, focusing on older adults, has explicitly sought to examine the relationship between pet ownership and health by testing explanatory models using eating habits and physical activity as the possible mechanisms. In this cross-sectional study of 127 elderly adults 60 years of age and older, Dembicki and colleagues (1996) found that pet owners had significantly lower serum triglycerides than non-pet owners and the dog owners walked significantly longer than non-pet owners and cat owners. Although these findings are compelling, the authors stated that the differences observed between pet owners and non-pet owners with respect to serum triglyceride levels could not be explained by physical activity. While these cross-sectional results show that pet ownership is associated with improved health status, it is still unknown whether pets cause people to be healthier, or if healthier people choose to own pets.

Longitudinal studies provide better evidence about the causal link between pet ownership and improved overall health. Some of these studies have also proposed that increased physical activity could be a possible explanation for this relationship. In 1991, Serpell conducted a 10-month longitudinal study examining changes in physical health, psychological health, and exercise levels of 71 adult subjects who recently acquired a pet (47 dog owners and 24 cat owners) compared with 26 non-pet owners. In this study, dog owners increased their walking more over a 10-month period following pet acquisition than non-pet owners. Moreover, dog owners reported a significant reduction in minor health problems, psychological components of ill-health (i.e., General Health Questionnaire [GHQ] scores), and increased their frequency and duration of recreational walking compared with cat owners. Non-pet owners did not report a significant change in the number of minor health problems or demonstrate a change in GHQ scores, but they did significantly increase their walking over the 10-month study period. Serpell noted that increased physical activity among dog owners could have long-term health implications and that the results highlighted that dogs and cats have different impacts on their owners' health.

In a prospective study of 1,054 Canadians 65 years of age and older, pet owners were younger, currently married living with someone, and more physically active compared to non-pet owners (Raina, Waltner-Toews, Bonnett, Woodward, & Abernathy, 1999). Moreover, pet owners had significantly higher activities of daily living (ADL) scores (i.e., higher scores indicating better health than non-pet owners over the one year period). In fact, ADL levels of non-pet owners deteriorated significantly more, on average, than pet owners. The authors reported that physical activity may be the reason for the relationship between pet owners and ADLs. Other likely reasons may be due to the pet owners being younger, more physically active, and thus able to perform their activities of daily living.

Each of these studies found that pet ownership, especially dog ownership, was associated with both increased physical activity and improved health. However, while these studies suggest that physical activity could be a possible mechanism by which pet ownership could lead to improved health, it is clear from these studies that more specific models need to be tested to determine if increased physical activity can explain the association between pet ownership and improved health in older adults. These findings may be particularly important for the older population where decreased physical activity is associated with increased disability, morbidity, and mortality.

The findings from studies that have examined the relationship between pet ownership and physical activity (Anderson et al., 1992; Bauman et al., 2001; Dembicki & Anderson, 1996; Headey, 1999; Raina et al., 1999; Serpell, 1991) indicate that dog owners are more physically active and more likely to meet the recommended level of physical activity than non-dog owners. Because physical activity levels appear to differ for dog and cat owners, it is possible that there will be some differences in the health status of dog and cat owners. If dog owners are more likely to exercise than non-pet or cat owners, then one would expect dog owners to have an improved health status, particularly cardiovascular health. In other words, it is possible that physical activity could be a mechanism by which pets, specifically dogs, confer health benefits. However, no studies have been able to clearly demonstrate that improved health is specifically mediated through increased dog-related physical activity. Figure 5.1 displays the conceptual model of the relationship between dog ownership, physical activity, and human health. Specifically, we posit that physical activity facilitated through dog walking confers improvements in health. Studies are needed to clearly illustrate the relationship between dog ownership and physical activity in older adults and the effect this has on the physical, psychological, and emotional health of older adults.

Figure 5.1. Conceptual model of dog ownership, physical activity, and health.

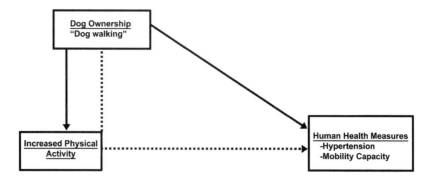

This model depicts dog ownership as being associated not only with improved health, but also with increased physical activity, and it is increased physical activity facilitated through dog walking that confers improvements in health.

Thorpe and colleagues used data from the Health, Aging, and Body Composition (Health ABC) study to examine the relationship between pet/dog ownership and human health (Thorpe et al., 2006; Thorpe, 2004). This study had a number of methodological strengths: 1) it included longitudinal data on the relationship between pet/dog ownership, physical activity, and health among older adults; 2) the sample included well-functioning older adults (70 to 79 years old at year 1); 3) the data included objective clinical measurements as well as self-reported data; 4) a number of measures of physical activity were collected; 5) additional information on participant health behaviors, physical function, cognitive function, hospitalization, and pet ownership status was collected; and 6) it provided an opportunity to test an explanatory model—increased physical activity as an explanation of the relationship between dog ownership and hypertension and mobility.

The results of this study showed that dog owners had a greater frequency and longer duration of casual walks than non-pet and non-dog owners (Thorpe et al., 2006). Further, while increased physical activity was associated with decreased prevalence of hypertension, physical activity among cat or dog owners did not significantly influence the relationship between pet ownership and hypertension. Thus, this study provided no statistical evidence of an association between pet ownership, physical activity, and prevalence or recent onset of hypertension in a population of older adults (Thorpe, 2004). In a subsequent analysis of this data, Thorpe and colleagues found that dog walking facilitated the achievement of prescribed weekly goals for physical activity and that this was associated with faster gait speed, a mobility advantage that was maintained over three years relative to non-dog walkers (Thorpe et al., 2006). Gait speed is the amount of time to walk over a short distance and is a predictor of independence in older adults. However, the results suggest that in older adults, dog walking may not be sufficient enough to impact the rate of decline in mobility among older adults.

Future directions for dog walking and physical activity in older adults

While these findings have added to the burgeoning HAI literature, additional work is still needed to completely understand the link between dog walking, physical activity, and human health, particularly in older adults. To advance the field of HAI research, future studies now need to move beyond cross-sectional analyses and include prospective, observational studies with robust study designs. For example, adequate sample sizes of dog owners and dog

walkers should be obtained as well as asking the same battery of dog ownership and dog walking questions each round of data collection. Intervention
research is also needed for older adults to determine if they would become
more physically active if provided a dog or access to a dog. Pet-specific studies
need to be conducted, or at least different types of pets and their relationship
with physical activity and health need to be clearly identified and analyzed in
studies. Furthermore, the extent to which the relationship between pet ownership and health varies by race or socioeconomic status (SES) requires further
investigation as minorities and members of low SES groups consistently exhibit higher rates of negative health behaviors, morbidity, and mortality. With
the increased proportion of aged minorities and magnitude of the race- and
SES-related differences in health outcomes, understanding the role of pets by
social stratifications for a better quality of life should be a high priority. These
efforts will provide key information necessary for health promoting strategies
and interventions that may ultimately lead to policies.

Conclusion

In summary, understanding the relationship between dog ownership, physical activity, and human health in older adults is in its infancy. With further
well-designed longitudinal and intervention studies the field of HAI will be
advanced, and this will lead to a body of evidence that will guide public health
policy and practice to positively impact population health. Hopefully, at that
time pets, specifically dogs, will be seen as having the ability to modify lifestyle behaviors and thus enhance our health

References

American Pet Products Manufacturers Association. (2009). *2009/2010
APPMA national pet owners survey*. Greenwich, CT: American Pet Products
Manufacturers Association, Inc.

Andersen, L. B., Schnohr, P., Schroll, M., & Hein, H. O. (2000). All-cause
mortality associated with physical activity during leisure time, work, sports,
and cycling to work. *Archives of Internal Medicine, 160*(11), 1621-1628.

Anderson, W. P., Reid, C. M., & Jennings, G. L. (1992). Pet ownership and risk
factors for cardiovascular disease. *Medical Journal of Australia, 157*(5), 298-301.

Bauman, A. E., Russell, S. J., Furber, S. E., & Dobson, A. J. (2001). The
epidemiology of dog walking: An unmet need for human and canine health.
Medical Journal of Australia, 175(11-12), 632-634.

Berkman, L. F., Berkman, C. S., Kasl, S., Freeman, D. H., Leo, L., Ostfeld, A. M., Cornoni-Huntley, J., & Brody, J. A. (1986). Depressive symptoms in relation to physical health and functioning in the elderly. *American Journal of Epidemiology, 124*, 372-388.

Berlin, J. A., & Colditz, G. A. (1990). A meta-analysis of physical activity in the prevention of coronary heart disease. *American Journal of Epidemiology, 132*(4), 612-28.

Boldt, M., & Dellmann-Jenkins, M. (1992). The impact of companion animals in later life and considerations for practice. *Journal of Applied Gerontology, 11*(2), 228-239.

Branch, L. G., & Jette, A. M. (1981). The Framingham disability study: I. social disability among the aging. *American Journal of Public Health, 71*, 1202-1210.

Chobanian, A. V., Bakris, G. L., Black, H. R., Cushman, W. C., Green, L. A., Izzo, J. L. Jr, Jones, D. W., Paterson, B. J., Peril, S., Wright, J. T. Jr, Rochelle, E. J., Joint National Committee on Prevention, Detection, Evaluation, and Treatment of High Blood Pressure. National Heart, Lung, and Blood Institute & National High Blood Pressure Education Program Coordinating Committee. (2003). Seventh report of the joint national committee on prevention, detection, evaluation, and treatment of high blood pressure. *Hypertension, 42*(6), 1206-1252.

Clark, D. O. (1996). The effect of walking on lower body disability among older blacks and whites. *American Journal of Public Health, 86*(1), 57-61.

Dembicki, D. (1995). *Association of pet ownership with eating, exercise, nutritional status, and heart health of seniors.* Unpublished, Colorado State University, Department of Food Science and Human Nutrition, Fort Collins, CO.

Dembicki, D., & Anderson, J. (1996). Pet ownership may be a factor in improved health of the elderly. *Journal of Nutrition for the Elderly, 15*(3), 15-31.

Estes, E. H., Jr. (1969). Health experiences in the elderly. In E. W. Buses & E. Pfeiffer (Eds.), *Behavior and adaptation in late life.* Boston: Little, Brown.

Ferrucci, L., Izmirlian, G., Leveille, S., Phillips, C. L., Corti, M. C., Brock, D. B., & Gurnalik, J. M. (1999). Smoking, physical activity, and active life expectancy. *American Journal of Epidemiology, 149*(7), 645-653.

Garrity, T. F., Stallones, L., Marx, M., & Johnson, T. (1989). Pet ownership and attachment as supportive factors in the health of the elderly. *Anthrozoos, 3*(1), 35-44.

Gillum, R. F., & Obisesan, T. O. (2010). Physical activity, cognitive function, and mortality in a US national cohort. *Annals of Epidemiology, 20*(4), 251-257.

Gregg, E. W., Pereira, M. A., & Caspersen, C. J. (2000). Physical activity, falls, and fractures among older adults: A review of the epidemiologic evidence. *Journal of the American Geriatrics Society, 48*(8), 883-893.

Hakim, A., Petrovitch, H., Burchfiel, C., Ross, G., Rodriguez, B., White, L., Yano, K., Curb, J., & Abbott, R. (1998). Effects of walking on mortality among nonsmoking retired men. *New England Journal of Medicine, 338*, 94-99.

Headey, B. (1999). Health benefits and health cost savings due to pets: Preliminary estimates from an Australian national survey. *Social Indicators Research, 47*(2), 233-243.

Heesch, K. C., Byles, J. E., & Brown, W. J. (2008). Prospective association between physical activity and falls in community-dwelling older women. *Journal of Epidemiology and Community Health, 62*(5), 421-426.

Houde, S. C., & Melilo, K. D. (2002). Cardiovascular health and physical activity in older adults: An integrative review of research methodology and results. *Journal of Advanced Nursing, 38*(3), 219-234.

Jette, A. M., & Branch, L. G. (1981). The Framingham disability study: II. physical disability among the aging. *American Journal of Public Health, 71*, 1211-1216.

Katcher, A. H. (1982). Are companion animals good for your health? A review of evidence. *Aging, 31-332*, 2-8.

Koenig, H., Hays, J., & Larson, D. (1999). Does religious attendance prolong survival? A six-year follow-up study of 3,968 older adults. *Journal of Gerontology: Medical Sciences, 54*, M370-376.

Laforest, S., Pelletier, A., Gauvin, L., Robitaille, Y., Fournier, M., Corriveau, H., & Filiatrault, J. (2009). Impact of a community-based falls prevention program on maintenance of physical activity among older adults. *Journal of Aging and Health, 21*(3), 480-500.

Lago, D., Delaney, M., Miller, M., & Grill, C. (1989). Companion animals, attitudes toward pets, and health outcome among the elderly: A long-term follow-up. *Anthrozoos, 331-332*(1), 25-34.

Lautenschlager, N. T., Cox, K. L., Flicker, L., Foster, J. K., van Bockmeer, F. M., Xiao, J., Greenop, K. R., & Almeida, O. P. (2008). Effect of physical activity on cognitive function in older adults at risk for Alzheimer's disease: A randomized trial. *Journal of the American Medical Association, 300*(9), 1027-1037.

Marx, M. B., Stallones, L., & Garrity, T. F. (1987). Demographics of pet ownership among U.S. elderly. *Anthrozoos, 1*, 36-40.

Mendes de Leon, C. F., Glass, T. A., & Berkman, L. F. (2003). Social engagement and disability in a community population of older adults. *American Journal of Epidemiology, 157*(7), 633-642.

Mensink, G. B. M., Ziese, T., & Kok, F. J. (1999). Benefits of leisure-time physical activity on the cardiovascular risk profile at older age. *International Journal of Epidemiology, 28*, 659-666.

Murrell, S. A., Himmelfarb, S., & Wright, K. (1983). Prevalence of depression and its correlates in older adults. *American Journal of Epidemiology, 117*, 173-185.

Musick, M. A., Herzog, A. R., & House, J. S. (1999). Volunteering and mortality among older adults: Findings from a national sample. *Journal of Gerontology: Social Sciences, 54*(3), S173-180.

National Institutes of Health. (1988). *Health benefits of pets*. DHHS Publication No. 1988-216-107. Washington, DC: U.S. Government Printing Office.

Ory, M., & Goldberg, E. (1983). Pet possession and life satisfaction in elderly women. In A. H. Katcher & A. M. Beck (Eds.), *New perspectives on our lives with companion animals* (pp. 803-817). Philadelphia: University of Pennsylvania Press.

Powell, K. E., Thompson, P. D., Caspersen, C. J., & Kendrick, J. S. (1987). Physical activity and the incidence of coronary heart disease. *Annual Review of Public Health, 8*(253), 87.

Raina, P., Waltner-Toews, D., Bonnett, B., Woodward, C., & Abernathy, T. (1999). Influence of companion animals on the physical and psychological health of older people: An analysis of a one-year longitudinal study. *Journal of the American Geriatrics Society, 47*(3), 323-329.

Rauramaa, R., Vaisanen, S. B., Rankinen, T., Penttila, I. M., Saarikoski, S., Tuomilehto, J., & Nissinen, A. (1995). Inverse relation of physical activity and apolipoprotein AI to blood pressure in elderly women. *Medicine and Science in Sports and Exercise, 27*, 164-169.

Robb, S. S., & Stegman, C. E. (1983). Companion animals and elderly people: A challenge for evaluators of social support. *Gerontologist, 23*(3), 277-282.

Rowan, A. N. (1991). Editorial: Do companion animals provide a health benefit? *Anthrozoos, 4*, 212-213.

Serpell, J. (1991). Beneficial effects of pet ownership on some aspects of human health and behaviour. *Journal of the Royal Society of Medicine, 84*(12), 717-720.

Siegel, J. (1990). Stressful life events and use of physician services among the elderly: The moderating role of pet ownership. *Journal of Personality and Social Psychology, 58*(6), 1081-1086.

Siegel, J. (1993). Companion animals: In sickness and in health. *Journal of Social Issues, 49*(1), 157-167.

Simonsick, E. M., Lafferty, M. E., Phillips, C. L., Mendes de Leon, C. F., Kasl, S. V., Seeman, T. E., Fillenbaum, G., Hebert, P., & Lemke, J. H. (1993). Risk due to inactivity in physically capable older adults. *American Journal of Public Health, 83*, 1443-1450.

Stallones, L., Marx, M., Garrity, T., & Johnson, T. (1990). Pet ownership and attachment in relation to the health of U.S. adults 21 to 64 years of age. *Anthrozoos, 4*(2), 100-112.

Tanaka, H., Reiling, M. J., & Seals, D. R. (1998). Regular walking increases peak limb vasodilatory capacity of older hypertensive humans: Implications for arterial structure. *Journal of Hypertension, 16*, 423-428.

Thorpe, R. J., Jr., Kreisle, R. A., Glickman, L. T., Simonsick, E. M., Newman, A. B., & Kritchevsky, S. (2006). Relationship between physical activity and pet ownership in year 3 of the Health ABC Study. *Journal of Aging and Physical Activity, 14*(2), 154-169.

Thorpe, R. J., Jr. (2004). Relationships between pet ownership, physical activity, and human health among elderly persons. (Doctoral dissertation) Purdue University, Indiana.

U.S. Department of Health and Human Services. (1999). Exercise: A guide from the national institute on aging (pp. 6). Bethesda, MD: National Institute on Aging, National Institutes of Health.

U.S. Department of Health and Human Services. (1996). *Physical activity and health: A report of the surgeon general.* No. S/N 017-023-00196-5. Atlanta, GA: U. S. Department of Health and Human Services, Centers for Disease Control and Prevention, National Center for Chronic Disease Prevention and Health Promotion.

U.S. Department of Health and Human Services. (2001). *Healthy People 2010.* Washington, DC: US Department of Health and Human Services.

Weih, M., Abu-Omar, K., Esselmann, H., Gelbrich, G., Lewczuk, P., Rutten, A., Wiltfang, J., & Kornhuber, J. (2009). Physical activity and prevention of Alzheimer's dementia: Current evidence and feasibility of an intervention trial. *Fortschritte Der Neurologie-Psychiatrie, 77*(3), 146-151.

Williamson, J. D., Espeland, M., Kritchevsky, S. B., Newman, A. B., King, A. C., Pahor, M., Guralnik, J. M., Pruitt, L. A., Miller, M. E., & LIFE Study Investigators. (2009). Changes in cognitive function in a randomized trial of physical activity: Results of the lifestyle interventions and independence for elder pilot study. *Journals of Gerontology. Series A, Biological Sciences and Medical Sciences, 64*(6), 688-694.

Chapter 6

"Walk a hound, lose a pound": A community dog walking program for families

Rebecca A. Johnson and Charlotte A. McKenney

Obesity and physical activity

It is estimated that obesity and overweight-attributable illness cost $1.6 bil-lion in medical expenditures in the state of Missouri alone between 1998 and 2000 (Finkelstein et al., 2004). Similar trends have been noted in the rest of the U.S. and other industrialized nations. Rising rates of obesity have been linked with the problem of limited physical activity (PA). Obesity is a key component of metabolic syndrome, a precursor to several chronic illnesses (including diabetes) and also to decline in physical functioning. These are major problems as people age, because accrual of obesity-related illnesses oc-curs to the point that by the time adults reach retirement, many have four or more chronic illnesses. Thus there is heightened attention to the obesity and overweight epidemic and the need for action to slow or stop it, subsequently preventing accrual of these illnesses.

The U.S. Department of Health and Human Service's Healthy People 2010 report called for adults of any age to engage in at least 30 minutes and children to engage in at least 60 minutes of moderate PA on most days or pref-erably every day (2000; DHHS, 2008), and the U.S. Surgeon General's call in 2001 was that society take a public health approach to changing citizens' lifestyles to increase PA. The extensive worldwide and personal consequences of obesity and physical inactivity-related health problems have focused the ur-gent need for effective interventions to increase total daily PA. However, PA and exercise programs found in the research literature have reported limited success in obesity prevention and weight maintenance.

Benefits of physical activity

There is general agreement in the literature that exercise can lead to a 1% to 4% loss of body fat (ACSM Position Stand, 1998). Body Mass Index (BMI) and weight loss are important predictors of health status (Doll, Petersen, & Stewart-Brown, 2000; Stafford, Hemingway, & Marmot, 1998). Weight loss is essential if devastating chronic diseases such as hypertension, diabetes, and cardiovascular disease are to be prevented or quelled. Higher BMI and lower PA were associated with greater post-exercise heart rate response and recovery. PA and reduced BMI have been associated with lowered coronary artery disease risk (Powell & Blair, 1994), better skeletal muscle metabolism (Suominen, Heikkinen, Liesen, Michel, & Hollman, 1977), pulmonary function (Wong, Wong, Pang, Azizah, & Dass, 2003), reduced mortality across genders (Barlow, Kohl, Gibbons, & Blair, 1995; Blair, Kohl, Paffenbarger, Clark, Cooper, & Gibbons, 1989), and improved natural killer cell activity (McFarlin, Flynn, Phillips, Stewart, & Timmerman, 2005). Evidence suggests that those in middle age (50 to 60 years) can have significantly lowered risk of major health problems due to chronic disease if they engage in regular exercise, and that even moderate-intensity physical activity improved aerobic fitness (Duscha et al., 2005). These findings held even if participants were obese (He & Baker, 2004). In fact, one group of investigators reported that men who had the lowest physical activity levels in their five-year study showed substantial benefits in preventing weight gain through increasing physical activity (Di Pietro, Dziura, & Blair, 2004). There is evidence that this benefit extends to women. Hills, Byrne, Wearing, & Armstrong, (2006) found that in obese men and women, "walking for pleasure" generated heart rates sufficient to improve cardiovascular fitness.

Despite the health benefits, less than one-third of adults of any age engage in recommended levels of PA for health benefits. A need exists for effective, evidence-based, sustainable strategies to increase regular participation in PA. An association appears to exist between community service or volunteer activities and levels of PA. Data from the 1998-1999 Greenstyles volunteer survey indicated that individuals who volunteered were more likely to meet PA recommendations than non-volunteers, and that those who volunteered in environmental activities (e.g., those that require PA) were 2.6 times as likely to meet PA recommendations as those who did not volunteer for these activities

(Librett et al., 2005). Thus, if PA is associated with volunteerism, there may be better likelihood of adherence and positive outcomes. People may be especially likely to participate in PA if it involves volunteering for a worthy cause, and especially if it includes an element of fun (Zeltzman & Johnson, 2011).

Benefits of dog walking

There is initial empirical support for using dogs as beneficial components of a walking protocol; however, studies have largely involved older adults. For example, Motooka, Koike, Yokoyama, & Kennedy (2006) found that when older adults walked with a dog, they had significantly greater parasympathetic nervous system activity (high frequency power heart rate variability) than when they walked without a dog. Other investigators found that even older adults who walked their dogs were more likely to achieve optimal activity levels per week and had faster usual and rapid walking speeds than those who did not walk their dogs (Thorpe et al., 2006b). In another study, investigators found that older adult dog owners engaged in more PA than did non-dog owners (Thorpe et al., 2006a).

Epidemiological evidence has suggested that dog walking (in a dog ownership context) may be an effective mechanism for increasing PA. In Australia, dog owners walked 18 minutes per week more than non-dog owners and were more likely to meet PA recommendations of 150 minutes per week (Bauman et al., 2000). A study in the United Kingdom found that dog owners accumulated significantly more exercise than either cat owners or adults without pets (Serpell, 1991). Further, data from the U.S. National Household Travel Survey revealed that nearly half of adults who walked dogs in the United States in 2001 accumulated at least 30 minutes of walking in bouts of at least 10 minutes (Ham & Epping, 2006). Additionally, an intervention trial in the U.S. found that obese individuals with pets increased their moderate physical activity over that of obese individuals without pets, and that the majority of the increase in moderate physical activity in the pet owners was obtained by engaging in dog-related activities (Kushner et al., 2006). These findings relate to dog owners' commitment to their animals' PA.

However, these studies only tell us the benefits of walking with one's own dog. The "Walk a Hound, Lose a Pound" (WAHLAP) program is an innovative and original contribution to the literature as the first study in which participants walk with shelter dogs. In this context, the social support provided by the dog may meet the criterion of Stahl et al. (2001) in which the social environment was a strong predictor of physical activity and fostered group cohesion (Estabrooks, 2000). The dog may be a social lubricant for participants and their families to communicate while walking and afterward. Wing and Jeffery (1999) found that providing a strong social component in a physical activity program decreased attrition. One study suggests that people can commit to regularly walking dogs that they do not own, and in the process, significantly increase their own PA (Johnson & Meadows, 2010).

Dog walking may have potential for improving long-term PA adherence through increasing readiness to engage in PA even beyond the dog walking. Readiness has been the most consistently identified correlate of PA adherence, and randomized, controlled trials have demonstrated that participants who exercised more frequently enjoyed the activity in which they engaged, received greater social support, and tended to maintain PA participation beyond termination of the intervention (McAuley et al., 2003). Dog walking may provide social support and enjoyment from which PA readiness can be increased, and long-term PA adherence stimulated.

One reason proposed for low rates of long-term adherence to PA is that typical programs do not promote purposeful activity (Morgan, 2001). The significance of purposeful PA in long-term adherence was demonstrated in 10 case studies of individuals who regularly participated in PA for periods ranging from 5 to 79 years. In seven of the case studies, individuals walked either for transportation or to walk a dog. In three cases, individuals walked dogs, and those individuals reported walking 3 to 6 miles per day, a minimum of five days per week, for periods ranging from 5 to 15 years. These levels of sustained PA meet or surpass current public health PA recommendations. Participants reported that the reason for their regular adherence was due to the need to exercise the dog (Morgan, 2001).

Based on its potential for increasing PA frequency, enjoyment, and adherence, as well as providing social support and purposeful PA, dog walking may increase PA readiness. If dog walking can induce sustained PA and facilitate readiness for participants to engage in additional PA outside of the dog walking, then we may make a significant contribution to preventing or decreasing an overweight and obese population.

Theoretical framework

The study was formulated on theoretical notions that converge around the concept of physical activity behavior change. Some of the constructs delineated in the Transtheoretical Model (TTM) may predict and explain participants' intention to begin and adhere to PA (Prochaska & DiClemente, 1982; Prochaska,

Redding, & Evers, 2002). A central concept of the model, which guided the present study, was stages of change (the intention and motivation to change). The stages of change related to physical activity are precontemplation (person has no intention of engaging in physical activity), contemplation (person has been thinking about starting physical activity in the near future, but not yet doing so), action (person is doing some physical activity), and maintenance (person is sustaining physical activity levels [e.g. 20 minutes, 3 times per week]). Investigators have applied and tested the TTM in the context of physical activity behavior change in several studies and reported that it was effective in predicting and explaining this behavior (Cardinal, Kosma, & McCubbin, 2004; Marcus, Rakowski, & Rossi, 1992; Marcus, Rossi, Selby, Niaura, & Abrams, 1992; Marcus, Selby, Niaura, & Rossi, 1992; Marcus & Simkin, 1993; Purath, Miller, McCabe, & Wilbur, 2004).

Behavioral processes of change facilitate or impede the change. They have been referred to as barriers and facilitators of the change—in this case walking—that may make the transition from precontemplation to action either more of a burden and less likely, or more positive and likely. Barriers to exercise have been reported, including convenience, transportation, cost, lack of proper equipment, lack of skill, inclement weather, concern about safety of the physical activity, and concern about unsafe neighborhoods in which to be physically active or go to and from exercise (Brawley, Rejeski, & King, 2003). Facilitators include simple programs that are convenient, inexpensive, and include a component of social support.

The dog walking model consists of several theoretical principles. First, there is the notion that the attractiveness of walking with a dog (facilitator of change) will be a major factor in the participants' decision to move through the stages of change to the action stage where they begin walking. Next, is the premise that the dog walking program addresses multiple barriers to exercise (such as cost—low charge to participants; convenience—location is easy to reach; safety—walking is an activity with low-risk of injury; skills needed to succeed—walking requires no special skills; and safety of neighborhoods—participants walk with shelter dogs near the animal shelter). Next, the intervention includes walking facilitators such as unconditional social support of the dog, identification with the study through T-shirts with the study logo, frequent contact with study staff, and convenience of walks at the animal shelter (Eyler, Brownson, Bacak, & Housemann, 2003). The dog walking model also provides self-monitoring of progress via the "Dog Walking Worksheets" and regular data collection. According to the TTM, taking all of these measures into account should predict beneficial outcomes from the dog walking intervention.

From a public health point of view, the logic model created by Epping (2003) was a useful guide in operationalizing the study. Essentially, it construes a sequence of developing a community-based study so that structures are put in place to ensure the sustainability of the WAHLAP program after the study is completed. A common criticism of community-based research is that useful programs are started, their efficacy tested, and when the funding ends, the program ends. To prevent this, WAHLAP was developed according to the logic model in Figure 6.1. The collaborative nature of the program helps to facilitate sustainability because more than one agency or entity is vested in its success. Toward that end, WAHLAP aimed to facilitate PA in human participants while providing needed exercise for the shelter dogs.

Figure 6.1. WAHLAP logic model.

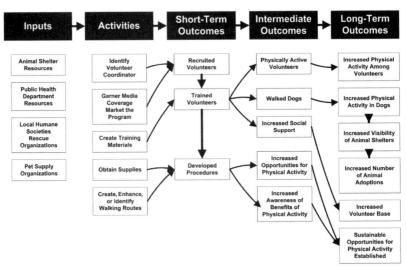

The purpose of the one-group, pretest-posttest study reported herein was to ascertain to what extent participating in a community dog walking program was associated with increased PA readiness, weight loss, and PA outside of the walking program.

Design and method

Participant recruitment

The study was advertised through various media outlets as part of a collaboration between the Research Center for Human-Animal Interaction, the State Department of Health and Senior Services, the local Parks and Recreation Department, and the local Humane Society animal shelter. Promotions included newspaper ads, radio and television interviews, and fliers posted in human and veterinary medical clinics, pet supply stores, and fitness facilities. Additionally, a video advertisement was broadcast periodically over the city cable television channel, and the program was announced in the weekly community calendar at a local affiliate network television channel.

The study was approved by the University of Missouri Health Sciences Institutional Review Board. Adults who could commit to four weeks of participation and were age 18 years or older were eligible to participate. Prospective participants came to the study site (Humane Society animal shelter), received an explanation of the study, and signed consent forms.

Data collection

Table 6.1 shows the data collection plan. Participants completed baseline, weekly, and final data collection (at four weeks) at the study site.

Table 6.1. Data collection plan.

Variable	Baseline	Weekly	Four Weeks
Demographic Information	X		
Pet Ownership History	X		
Health History	X		
Height	X		
Weight/BMI	X	X	X
Blood Pressure	X	X	X
PA Stage of Change	X		X
7-Day PA Recall	X	X	X
Program Perceptions			X
Attendance		X	

Instruments

The PA "stage of change" instrument comprises a list of eight statements, each delineating a more advanced stage of change in the participant's PA status (Prochaska & DiClemente, 1982). PA readiness is classified as precontemplation, contemplation, preparation, action, or maintenance. The items range from 1) "I don't do regular vigorous or moderate exercise now, and I don't intend to start in the next 6 months" to 8) "I've been doing vigorous exercise 3 or more days per week for the last 6 months or more." The participants completed this instrument at baseline and after four weeks of participation.

The 7-Day Physical Activity Record covered PA for the week including the day of participation in the WAHLAP program and was completed by participants (Table 6.2). The instrument was based on recall and was investigator-developed. Frequencies of the activities were summed and compared from baseline to four week counts.

Table 6.2. Seven-day physical activity record.
How often did you exercise in the past week that caused you break into a sweat?
Please write the number of times each week beside the activity
that you did.

	Activity performed	Number of times each week
1.	Stretching	
2.	Walking	
3.	Running	
4.	Free-weight lifting	
5.	Weight machines	
6.	Treadmill	
7.	Stepper machine	
8.	Stationary bike	
9.	Elliptical machine	
10.	Other (please specify)	
11.	Other (please specify)	
12.	Other (please specify)	

Weight was recorded at each data collection point at the same time of day using the same scales. A Seca model 700 balance beam scale was used to obtain the height and weight. The height rod read from 24 inches to 78 inches. The weight capacity measured to 500 pounds. The base was a large, fan-shaped, cast-iron platform for increased stability and accuracy of measurement. Calibration of the scale was completed at the factory by company policy.

BMI (weight in kilograms divided by height in meters squared) was calculated automatically by the SAS computer system prior to data analysis using weekly weight measurements taken before the participants walked a dog.

Dog walking protocol

Each Saturday morning from 8 a.m. until 12 p.m., from April through October, community members came to the animal shelter to walk with shelter dogs. Participants preregistered through the Parks and Recreation Department's online or telephone registration system for one of three, one-hour time slots. They were welcomed by study staff and volunteers at the study home base, which consisted of an events tent with study signage and tables and located just outside of the animal shelter building.

Staff described the program to participants, obtained informed consent, and collected baseline data according to the data collection schedule (Table 6.1). Participants' blood pressure was measured by either a registered nurse or an undergraduate nursing student trained in blood pressure assessment technique, recognition of abnormal blood pressure levels, and procedures for addressing them. Participants whose blood pressure readings were higher than 150/90 (a level commonly recognized as needing attention of a health care provider) were prevented from walking and were recommended to contact their health care provider.

Educational pamphlets provided by the Missouri Department of Health and Senior Services including information on nutrition and physical activity were made available. Each participant received a WAHLAP T-shirt and the use of a fanny pack supplied with dog treats, a plastic bag designed for collecting dog refuse, and a card with emergency contact numbers.

Next, study staff led participants through a brief group warm-up exercise sequence including stretching exercises for the neck, shoulders, chest, and legs. Participants were given an explanation of safe dog and leash handling, and when necessary, a demonstration of how to use a dog refuse collection bag. Subsequently, participants selected a dog from those eligible for participation. Dog eligibility was determined by shelter staff who administered a standard behavior screening test. Participants chose a dog based on its size and exuberance compared with the participant's walking ability and other physical limitations.

Walking took place with other participants and study staff members on a shady gravel walking trail marked with WAHLAP mileage markers at 1/4 mile, 1/2 mile, 3/4 mile, and at the 1 mile with a sign denoting "turn around" to return to the shelter. A study staff member or volunteer carried a cellular telephone while patrolling the trail to ensure the safety of people and dogs. When participants had walked as far as they wanted to walk, they returned the dog to the study home base and signed out by responding to brief questions on their weekly data collection instrument about their experience while walking the dog. Bottled water was available at the home base for participants, as were water buckets for the dogs.

At their last walking session participants wrote responses to questions about why they chose to participate in the WAHLAP program, what they perceived as benefits of the WAHLAP program, what changes they would recommend, and why they continued their participation.

Findings

Sixty-nine participants completed the study. Table 6.3 shows their demographic characteristics. Weekly, from 10 to 30 dogs were walked. Participants reported "that it feels good being able to help the dogs get exercise, socialize with people and with dogs."

The sample was largely female and middle-aged with a median BMI level in the overweight category as determined by the National Heart Lung and Blood Institute of the National Institutes of Health (underweight=less than 18.5; normal weight=18.5-24.9; overweight=25-29.9; obese=over 30) (http://www.nhlbisupport.com/bmi/).

PA stage of change increased significantly over the four week study period (from 4.8 to 5.25), and there was a modest though statistically significant decrease in weight (three pounds). There was minimal change in BMI, which was statistically significant (Table 6.4). PA outside of the program did not significantly increase. Nor was PA stage of change significantly correlated with change in PA outside of the program (p=0.3807).

Discussion

Our findings show modest support for the notion that if people engage in a PA program that is socially supportive, purposeful, and beneficial to others, they may increase their PA readiness and be more likely to engage in other PA. Thus, maximizing the participants' perception of the walking protocol as socially supportive was important even beyond adherence to the protocol. Other investigators have reported that when participants feel support during the walking program, other physical activity has been show to increase

Table 6.3. Demographic findings (N=69).

Age		19 to 85 years	(Mean=43, SD=16.4)
Gender	Male	12	18%
	Female	57	82%
Married	Yes	38	55%
	No	31	45%
Education level	High school	26	38%
	College	43	62%
Race	Caucasian	64	93%
	African American	3	4%
	Asian	2	3%
Reported health problems	Mental health	20	(29%)
	Endocrine	11	(16%)
	Cardiovascular	10	(14%)
	Musculoskeletal	10	(14%)
	Cancer	2	(3%)
Pet owner	Yes	48	70%
	No	21	30%

Table 6.4. Physical activity, weight, and BMI findings (N=69).

Physical activity stage of change	Mean Pretest score=4.8	vigorous exercise < 3 times/week or moderate exercise < 5 times/week
	Mean Posttest score=5.25 (p=0.0013)	30 minutes/day of moderate exercise 5+days/month
Physical activity outside of program (n=59 with no missing data)	Median Pretest count=5	
	Median Posttest count=6	p=0.27
Weight	Pretest Posttest	Median=156 (SD=35, Range=98-250) Median=153 (SD=35, Range=100-245) p=0.0082*
BMI	Pretest Posttest	Median =26 (SD=4.4, Range=18-38) Median =25.8 (SD=4.4, Range=18-38) p=0.010*

*significant at p < 0.05

(Fiatarone et al., 1994). Through strong identification and interaction in the study (WAHLAP T-shirts worn weekly by participants, contact with study staff, opportunities to socialize with other people and with dogs), WAHLAP may be a community model for accomplishing the goals of enhancing PA and enhancing adoptability of shelter dogs.

Participants in the study regularly expressed joy at being able to help the shelter dogs get some exercise. This was consistent with findings of another study in which overweight, sedentary public housing residents had 72% adherence in a 52 week graduated intervention walking therapy dogs. These participants stated that their motivation for adherence was, "the dogs need us to walk them" (Johnson & Meadows, 2010).

In the present study, five participants completed volunteer training at the animal shelter to be able to walk the dogs more frequently outside of the study. Five participants adopted dogs that they had walked.

The project also served as an outlet for primary school-age children who came to walk shelter dogs with their parents and/or grandparents. Two of these children completed summer projects about dog walking for either their summer school classes or for a 4-H project (this resulted in an award). Fifty university students completed internships, clinical practica, volunteer experiences, or service learning projects through the WAHLAP program.

Shelter staff regularly commented that the shelter was a much quieter place and that the dogs "showed better" to potential adopters on Saturday afternoons after WAHLAP. This was an important outcome in that the greatest number of potential adopters of shelter dogs typically go to the shelter on Saturday afternoon. Additionally, during WAHLAP the dogs had regular socialization with other dogs and with people of all ages

Subsequently, in another study, the investigators tracked adoption and euthanasia rates in dogs participating in a graduated walking program with older adults and found that participating dogs were significantly more likely to be adopted and less likely to be euthanized than non-participating dogs (Johnson, McKenney, & McCune, 2010, unpublished).

The applicability of this small-scale study for use in population dog walking programs is high. The logic model used and procedures developed make the WAHLAP highly transportable to other communities wherever an animal shelter exists. Considering that the majority of cities in the U.S. and in many other countries have at least one animal shelter, it may be possible to implement a population-based WAHLAP initiative. Our participants found the WAHLAP program to be a fun endeavor in which they got some PA and helped the shelter animals in their community. This same logic may be readily applied to other populations, expanding dog walking from something that only dog owners can benefit from to something that all who are willing can enjoy.

Acknowledgments

The authors would like to acknowledge the support and assistance of the following:

Dr. Jack and Mrs. Vicki Stephens, the Skeeter Foundation, Dr. Joe and Mrs. Judy Roetheli, staff and volunteers of the Central Missouri Humane Society (especially Dr. Alan Allert, Patty Forister, and Heather Duren), staff and volunteers of the Columbia Parks and Recreation Department (especially Karen Ramey and Erin Carillo), and the Missouri Department of Health and Senior Services.

References

American College of Sports Medicine 1998: Position Stand. (1998). The recommended quantity and quality of exercise for developing and maintaining cardiorespiratory and muscular fitness, and flexibility in healthy adults. *Medicine and Science in Sports and Exercise. 30*, 975–991.

Barlow, C. E., Kohl, H. W., III, Gibbons, L. W., & Blair, S. N. (1995). Physical fitness, mortality and obesity. *International Journal of Obesity, 19*(Suppl. 4), S41-S44.

Bauman, A. E., Russell, S. J., Furber, S. E., & Dobson, A. J. (2000). The epidemiology of dog walking: An unmet need for human and canine health. *Medical Journal of Australia, 175*(11-12), 632-634.

Blair, S. N., Kohl, H. W., Paffenbarger, R. S., Jr., Clark, D. G., Cooper, K. H., & Gibbons, L. W. (1989). Physical fitness and all-cause mortality: A prospective study of healthy men and women. *Journal of the American Medical Association, 262*, 2395-2401.

Brawley, L. R., Rejeski, W. J., & King, A. C. (2003). Promoting PA for older adults: The challenges for changing behavior. *American Journal of Preventive Medicine, 25*(3Sii), 172-183.

Cardinal, B. J., Kosma, M., & McCubbin, J. A. (2004). Factors influencing the exercise behavior of adults with physical disabilities. *Medicine & Science in Sports & Exercise, 36*(5), 868-875.

Department of Defense. (2008). Defense Manpower Data Center, Contingency Tracking System files, data as of Dec. 31, 2008.

Di Pietro, L., Dziura, J., & Blair, S. N. (2004). Estimated change in physical activity level (PAL) and prediction of 5-year weight change in men: The Aerobics Center longitudinal study. *International Journal of Obesity, 28*(12), 1541-1547.

Doll, H., Petersen, S., & Stewart-Brown, S. (2000). Obesity and physical and emotional well-being: Associations between BMI, chronic illness and the physical and mental components of the SF-36. *Obesity Research, 8*(2), 160-170.

Duscha, B. D., Slentz, C. A., Johnson, J. L., Houmard, J. A., Bensimhon, D. R., Knetzger, K. J., & Kraus, W. E. (2005). Effects of exercise training amount and intensity on peak oxygen consumption in middle-age men and women at risk for cardiovascular disease. *Chest, 128*, 2788-2793.

Estabrooks, P. A. (2000). Sustaining exercise participation through group cohesion. *Exercise & Sport Sciences Reviews, 28*(2), 63-67.

Eyler, A. A., Brownson, R. C., Donatelle, R. J., King, A. C., Brown, D., & Sallis, J. F. (1999). PA, social support, and middle-and older-age minority women: Results from a U.S. survey. *Social Science Medicine, 49*, 781-789.

Finkelstein, E. A., Fiebelkorn, I. C., & Wang, G. (2004). State-level estimates of annual medical expenditures attributable to obesity. *Obesity Research, 12*(1), 18–24.

Ham S. A., & Epping, J. (2006). Dog walking and physical activity in the United States. *Preventing Chronic Disease, 3*(2), A47.

He, X. Z., & Baker, D. W. (2004). Body mass index, PA, and the risk of decline in overall health and physical functioning in late middle age. *American Journal of Public Health, 94*(9), 1567-1573.

Hills, A. P., Byrne, N. M., Wearing, S., & Armstrong, T. (2006). Validation of the intensity of walking for pleasure in obese adults. *Preventive Medicine, 42*(1), 47-50.

Johnson, R. A., McKenney, C., & McCune, S. (2010). Walk a hound, lose a pound and stay fit for seniors. Unpublished manuscript.

Johnson, R. A., & Meadows, R. L. (2010). Dog-walking: Motivation for adherence to a walking program. *Clinical Nursing Research, 19*(4), 387-402. DOI:10.1177/1054773810373122.

Kushner, R. F., Blatner, D. J., Jewell, D. E., & Rudloff, K. (2006). The PPET study: People and pets exercising together. *Obesity, 14*(10), 1762-1770.

Librett, J., Yore, M. M., Buchner, D. M., & Schmid, T. L. (2005). Take pride in America's health: Volunteering as a gateway to physical activity. *American Journal of Health Education, January/ February 36*(1).

Marcus, B. H, Rakowski, W., & Rossi, J. S. (1992). Assessing motivational readiness and decision making for exercise. *Health Psychology, 11*(4), 257-261.

Marcus, B. H, Selby, V. C., Niaura, R. S., & Rossi, J. S. (1992). Self-efficacy and the stages of exercise behavior change. *Research Quarterly for Exercise and Sport*, *63*(1), 60-66.

Marcus, B. H., & Simkin, L. R. (1993). The stages of exercise behavior. *The Journal of Sports Medicine and Physical Fitness*, *33*(1), 83-88.

Marcus, B. H., Rossi, J., S., Selby, V. C., Niaura, R. S., & Abrams, D. B. (1992). The stages and processes of exercise adoption and maintenance in a worksite sample. *Health Psychology*, *11*(6), 386-395.

McAuley, E. (1992). The role of efficacy cognitions in the prediction of exercise behavior in middle-aged adults. *Journal of Behavioral Medicine*, *15*(1), 65-88.

McFarlin, B. K., Flynn, M. G., Phillips, M. D. Stewart, L. K., & Timmerman, K. L. (2005). Chronic resistance exercise training improves natural killer cell activity in older women. *Journal of Gerontology A: Biological Science & Medical Science, October 1, 60*(10), 1315-1318.

Morgan, W. P. (2001). Prescription of physical activity: A paradigm shift. *Quest*, *53*(3), 366-382.

Motooka, M., Koike, H., Yokoyama, T., & Kennedy, N. (2006). Effect of dog-walking on autonomic nervous activity in senior citizens. *Medical Journal of Australia, 184*(2), 60-63.

Powell, K. E., & Blair, S. N. (1994). The public health burdens of sedentary living habits: Theoretical but realistic estimates. *Medicine and Science in Sports and Exercise, 26*(7), 851-856.

Prochaska, J. O., & DiClemente, C. C. (1982). Transtheoretical therapy: Toward a more integrative model of change. *Psychotherapy: Theory, Research & Practice*, *20*, 161-173.

Prochaska, J. O., Redding, C. A., & Evers, K. E. (2002). The transtheoretical model and stages of change. In K. Glanz, B. K. Rimer, & F. M. Lewis (Eds.), *Health behavior and health education, 3rd Ed.* (pp. 99-120). San Francisco, CA: Jossey-Bass.

Purath, J., Miller, A. M., McCabe, G., & Wilbur, J. (2004). A brief intervention to increase PA in sedentary working women. *Canadian Journal of Nursing Research*, *36*(1), 76-91.

Serpell, J. (1991). Beneficial effects of pet ownership on some aspects of human health and behaviour. *Journal of the Royal Society of Medicine*, *84*(12), 717-720.

Stahl, T., Rutten, A., & Nutbeam, D. (2001). The importance of the social environment for physically active lifestyle—results from an international study. *Social Science & Medicine, 52*(1), 1-10,

Suominen, H., Heikkinen, E., Liesen, H., Michel, D., & Hollman, W. (1977). Effects of 8 weeks' endurance training on skeletal muscle metabolism in 56-70 year-old sedentary men. *European Journal of Applied Physiology, 37*, 173-180.

Thorpe, R. J., Kreisle, R. A., Glickman, L. T., Simonsick, E. M., Newman, A. B., & Kritchevsky, S. (2006). Physical activity and pet ownership in year 3 of the Health ABC Study. *Journal of Aging and Physical Activity, 14*, 154-168.

Thorpe, R., J., Simonsick, E. M., Brach, J. S., Ayonayon, H., Satterfield, S., Harris, T. B., Garcia, M., & Kritchevsky, S. B. (2006). Dog ownership, walking behavior, and maintained mobility in late life. *Journal of the American Geriatric Society, 54*, 1419-1424.

Wing, R. R., & Jeffery, R. W. (1999). Benefits of recruiting participants with friends and increasing social support for weight loss and maintenance. *Journal of Consulting & Clinical Psychology. 67*(1), 132-138,

Wong, C. H., Wong, S. F., Pang, W. S., Azizah, M. Y., & Dass, M. J. (2003). Habitual walking and its correlation to better physical function: Implications for prevention of physical disability in older persons. *Journal of Gerontology A: Biological Science & Medical Science, 58*, 555-560.

Zeltzman, P., & Johnson, R. A. (2011). *Walk a hound, lose a pound: How you and your dog can lose weight, stay fit, and have fun together.* West Lafayette, IN: Purdue University Press.

Chapter 7

Method development and preliminary examination of dog walking as a form of human and canine physical activity

Barbour S. Warren, Joseph J. Wakshlag, Mary Maley, Tracy Farrell, Martin T. Wells, Angela M. Struble, Carol M. Devine, and Grace Long

Physical activity on a regular basis has been well documented to play an important role in weight control (Flegal Carroll, Ogden, & Curtin, 2010). Plus, there are numerous other health benefits that have been associated with regular physical activity. These include decreases in the risk of: heart disease, various types of cancer, diabetes, osteoporosis, and arthritis (Ogden, Yanovski, Carroll, & Flegal, 2007). In spite of these positive effects of physical activity, the most recent examinations have shown that 64% of Americans do not engage in the recommended levels of physical activity (Sapkota, Bowles, Ham, & Kohl, 2005). Worse yet, about 24% of the adult population report inactivity during their leisure time (Kruger, Ham, & Kohl, 2005). Lesser, but still elevated levels, for both these statistics were recently reported for youths in the 9th to 12th grades (34% and 6%, respectively) (Brener, Kann, Garcia, MacDonald, Ramsey, Honeycutt, Hawkins, Kinchens, & Harris, 2005).

Canine obesity has increased greatly in recent years in parallel to that in humans (German, 2006). Whereas 68% of humans are currently considered overweight or obese, nearly 40% of U.S. dogs are clinically diagnosed as overweight or obese (German, 2006). These changes also raise concern for the U.S. canine population as obesity in dogs has been associated with a spectrum of diseases similar to that observed in humans (German, 2006).

While obesity results from a complex interplay between genetics, behavior, and various aspects of an individual's environment, this disorder, in its most simple form, can be viewed as an imbalance between caloric intake and expenditure. Several studies have conducted human examinations into the size of the daily difference between caloric intake and expenditure, the so-called energy gap (Hill, Wyatt, Reed, & Peters, 2003; Hill, Peters, & Wyatt, 2009; Swinburn, Sacks, Lo, Westerterp, Rush, Rosenbaum, Luke, Schoeller, DeLany, Butte, & Ravussin, 2009). These studies have derived values close to a 50 kilocalorie daily excess. The small size of this difference has led to the suggestion that small changes in energy expenditure or intake carried out on a daily basis could be one strategy to address weight gain and the rise in obesity.

Physical activity directly reflects caloric expenditure and undoubtedly plays a critical role in the rise of overweight and obese citizens. Although there are numerous avenues of physical activity, walking provides a highly viable option. It is the most popular human (and likely canine/human) physical activity and is also inexpensive and convenient. Although walking has been promoted as a daily physical activity, little attention has been paid to dog ownership as a potentially important factor in its promotion. Dog walking has two key characteristics associated with sustained physical activity: purpose and social interaction. In line with being an activity with purpose, dog walking also favors regular daily participation for a period of reasonable time. These are critical characteristics as regular caloric expenditure is a highly feasible approach to closing the daily gap between caloric intake and expenditure.

Management of canine obesity, like that in humans, remains a major challenge requiring numerous approaches. Owner education does not hold great promise as recent studies have shown no lack of owner awareness and understanding related to overweight dogs (Yaissle, Holloway, & Buffington, 2004). While excessive calorie consumption is thought to play a dominant role in canine obesity, physical activity is likely to be a significant contributor, yet no direct correlation between obesity and physical activity has been derived in canine populations. Nonetheless, obesity management frequently includes a recommendation to increase physical activity. However, firm recommendations regarding the amount of activity needed to help address this growing problem have eluded both practitioners and academics.

Tools used to assess physical activity in canine and human studies include the use of physical activity questionnaires and motion detection devices such as pedometers and accelerometers (Chan, Spierenburg, Ihle, & Tudor-Locke, 2005; Laflamme, 2006). Some studies in humans suggest that use of accelerometers is preferable as the devices allow determination of physical activity intensity (Corder, Brage, & Ekelund, 2007). Yet in practice, especially in canine populations, this may not be practical as currently the cost is high and units tend to be sensitive to both positional placement and the type of activity (Westerterp, 1999). Although pedometers give no measure of activity intensity, they do provide an accurate, reliable, and inexpensive means of tracking walking volume. In addition, pedometers are highly adaptable as reflected by their use in studies of various species of animals including humans, dogs, cattle, horses, and turkeys (Chan et al., 2005; Hocking, Bernard, & Maxwell, 1999; Holland, Kronfeld, & Meacham, 1996; Mazrier, Tal, Aizinbud, & Bargai, 2006; Roelofs, van Eerdenburg, Soede, & Kemp, 2005).

The studies described in this chapter set out to develop and test tools and methodologies to examine the promotion of dog walking as a form of physical activity for both humans and canines. This chapter will first describe the development (Study 1), preliminary results in dogs (Study 2), and then detail some promising results in a group of human dog walkers (Study 3).

Results and discussion, study 1: Development of a pedometer-based method for measuring steps in dogs

The studies in this section aimed first to refine and validate a pedometer methodology for use in dogs and then to examine and compare typical physical activity in normal, overweight, and obese dogs.

Development of the pedometer methodology used 20 dogs of various sizes from 4.5 kg to 50 kg. These dogs were recruited from a companion animal clinic at the Cornell University Companion Animal Hospital and fitted with pedometer collars as shown in Figure 7.1. The collars consisted of a pedometer (Accusplit AE120 with a Yamax digiwalker engine or Accusplit 1120, Livermore, CA) suspended from an elastic bungee cord (3/8-inch diameter) using a threaded eye screw attached to the top of pedometer units. The eye screw was attached to the bungee cord collar using a small zip-locking cable tie. This configuration allowed the pedometer to hang in close to a vertical position and move freely, which was necessary for accurate counts. An adjustable collar loop was formed with the bungee cord by opposing each end using a larger zip-locking cable tie. This produced an apparatus that could be easily positioned for accuracy, put on, and taken off.

Validation of the accuracy and precision of the pedometer forefoot step counts focused on the trot gait. This gait was chosen as it is the most common gait for dogs, in general, and especially when they are walked on a leash. For evaluation, actual steps were determined by walking and videotaping dogs

Figure 7.1. Pedometer collar design. A pedometer (Accusplit AE120 with a Yamax digiwalker engine or Accusplit 1120, Livermore, CA) was modified and suspended from an elastic bungee cord and an adjustable zip tie to allow accurate positioning and easy on/off.

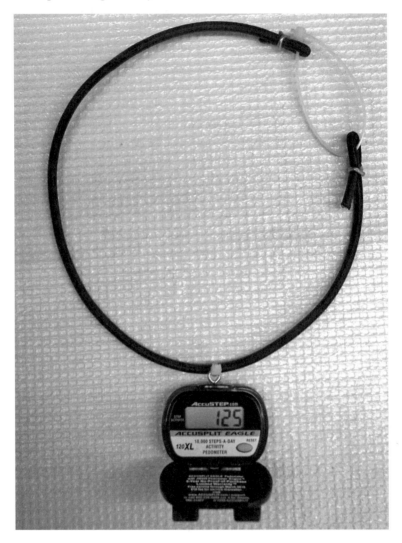

six times over a 25 m (82 ft) distance. There was a wide range of steps taken to cover this distance by the 20 differently sized dogs examined in this study. Steps ranged from 29 to 116, differing by a factor of 4. Accuracy of measured pedometer readings was determined by direct comparison of the actual steps counted on videotapes and those registered by the pedometers. Examination of the percentage difference between actual and measured step data revealed

Figure 7.2. Accuracy of pedometer design for dogs of different sizes. Dogs of various sizes were walked and videotaped six times over a 25 meter (82 ft) long distance. The pedometer readings were compared to the actual steps counted on videotapes by the percentage difference between the two values. Error bars indicate SEM.

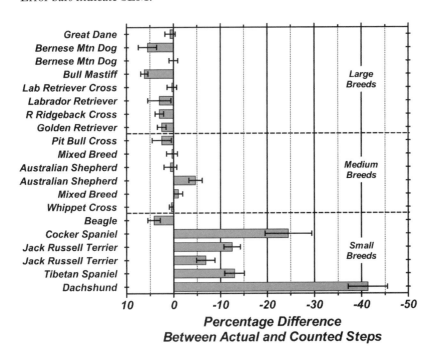

Percentage Difference
Between Actual and Counted Steps

that for only five dogs there was a considerable underestimation of the pedometer measured steps (Figure 7.2). All of these dogs weighed less than 10 kg and would be considered small. As a result of this finding, dogs were assessed as small, medium, and large size groups. The average percentage difference between actual (by videotape count) and measured steps was: -6.2% ± 1.3 for dogs of all sizes; -21.0% ± 3.0 for small sized dogs; -0.7 % ± 1.7 for medium sized dogs and 6.1% ± 1.3 for large sized dogs.[1] The mean difference between actual and pedometer measured steps for the medium and large sized dogs used in this part of the study was 3.3 % ± 1.2.

Dogs were also leash (1.8 m, 6 ft long) walked 3.2 km (2 mi) to assess the relative number of pedometer measured steps. The average number of steps taken in a 3.2 km walk was 6,056 ± 957 with a range of 4,737-7,135 steps.

The use of pedometers for assessing physical activity in dogs has previously been reported by Chan and colleagues (Chan et al., 2005). They examined a group of 26 dogs and reported that pedometers can be effectively used to determine daily walking activity in dogs. However, their methodology, using a lightweight chain collar, may not have been the best way to accurately utilize pedometers for dogs. This technique is contrary to design conditions for use in humans, which emphasize that pedometer accuracy depends on the unit being level in both the side to side and fore to aft planes. These are orientations that would allow accurate vertical swinging of the pedometer's counting pendulum. The Chan group's methodology reported an overall error of about a 15% difference between actual and counted steps for the walk/trot gait. The accurately lengthened bungee cord mounting technique allowed achievement of much greater overall accuracy for medium to large dogs, a difference of 3.3 ± 1.2%. Our newly developed methodology is not without its limitations as the accuracy in small dogs is much lower (difference = -21.0 ± 3%). However, examination of Figure 7.2 shows that the small dog value is heavily influenced by the very poor accuracy in one dachshund whose step difference exceeded 40%. Not including this outlying value produces accuracy values for the small dogs that are similar to those reported by the Chan group, although still greater than our method used in medium and large breeds.

Results and discussion, study 2: Assessment of walking steps among obese and non-obese dogs

The aim of this study was to assess dog walking activity among dogs of various sizes and body condition scores (BCS)[2] to inform the development of an intervention based on dog walking as a means of canine obesity prevention. In the general dog population only 10% of dogs may have BCS at obesity level values (8 and 9), while the majority of dogs will vary between 5 and 7. Consequently, the subpopulations in the extreme range of BCS values are rarely present in samples at numbers adequate for meaningful statistical representation (German, 2006). To address this issue, we recruited and oversampled an obese population of dogs. These 77 dogs were recruited either from an obesity clinic sample (OCS) (n=29 dogs) or a community-based dog walking project (CS) (n=48 dogs). Recruitment and pooling of these two groups allowed enrollment of a sufficient number of dogs with both high and normal BCS. The pooling produced a population that displayed a normal distribution of BCS centered on a value of 7 and ranged from 4 to 9 (data not shown).

The OCS was recruited as part of an obesity reduction protocol at the Cornell University Companion Animal Hospital in Ithaca, New York. This group was made up of overweight and obese dogs with BCS ranging from 7 to 9. Eligibility criteria included the 7 to 9 range of BCS and a medium to large size, defined as at least 36 cm (14 in) at the shoulder. Dog owners were instructed by the investigators on how to use pedometers and provided with a set of written instructions. In addition they were given a paper diary to note daily pedometer measured step counts of their dogs, during the first, sixth, and tenth weeks of a 10-week study period. Recruitment occurred throughout the 2008 calendar year. Owners were instructed that their dogs should wear the pedometers on walks or anytime they were physically active. They were also told not to use pedometers during any water-related activities. Only medium to large sized dogs were recruited because the methodology developed in Study 1 was most accurate in dogs this size. All dogs in the OCS were also given a therapeutic weight reduction food (Purina OM canned and dry diet, Nestlé-Purina, St. Louis, Missouri) and were encouraged to walk with their dogs. Dogs in the OCS had calorie restriction to achieve 1-1.5% weight loss per week. However, baseline BCS values were used for all analyses.

The second group of canine subjects, the CS, was recruited through the use of local newspaper and flier advertising in a rural community in Upstate New York. Participants were invited to join a wellness program involving dog walking. Dogs of 36 cm stature or larger were used again. There were no BCS limitations, but most dogs were in the 5 to 7 BCS range. This study used the same 10-week timeline with daily steps recorded on the first, sixth, and tenth weeks. In addition to the pedometer measured step counts among dogs, the owners of these dogs also wore pedometers during all waking hours and recorded both dog and human steps. Owners were instructed not to change theirs, or their dogs', current walking behavior. They were also instructed to record step counts either using a paper diary or a participant-specific, Web-based step log. As an incentive, owners of all dogs completing the study in this group were given coupons for a two-month supply of dog food (Nestlé-Purina, St. Louis, Missouri) and two general health examinations by a veterinarian. Table 7.1 lists the BCS and breed distribution of the pooled OCS and CS dogs. Their demographic characteristics are presented in Table 7.2.

Pooling the results of the OCS and CS samples allowed examination of the relationship between dog walking and BCS over a considerable range. The scatter plot shown in Figure 7.3 illustrates the relationship between the average number of daily steps during the three measurement weeks and baseline BCS. A Spearman's nonparametric regression analysis of these data revealed a significant correlation between the average daily step value over the course of the study and the baseline BCS (Spearman's rho=-0.5169, p-value < 0.0001). Higher daily steps were significantly associated with healthier baseline BCS. In addition, the average number of daily steps over the three separate weeks

Table 7.1. Dog breeds pooled from the OCS and CS groups and their BCS distribution. Numbers in parentheses indicate the number of individuals in each breed/BCS set.

Body Condition Score					
4	5	6	7	8	9
Australian Shepherd/ Chow Chow Cross (1)	Bassett Hound (2)	Border Collie (1)	Akita Cross (1)	Australian Shepherd (1)	Bernese Mountain Dog (2)
German Shepherd (1)	Boxer (1)	Beagle (1)	Border Collie/ Cocker Cross (1)	Beagle (3)	Bull Mastiff (1)
Great Dane Cross (1)	Golden Retriever (1)	Bulldog (1)	Beagle (1)	Bulldog (1)	Cocker Spaniel (1)
Husky/ Labrador Retriever Cross (1)	Labrador Retriever (1)	Doberman Pinscher (1)	Beagle/ Shepherd/B Collie Cross(1)	Labrador Retriever (5)	Golden Retriever (1)
	Labrador Retriever Cross (1)	English Setter (1)	Bernese Mountain Dog (1)	Mixed Breed (4)	Labrador Retriever (4)
	Schnauzer Poodle Cross (1)	Golden Retriever (1)	Boxer (1)	Siberian Husky (1)	Mixed Breed (1)
	Shepherd Collie Retriever Cross (2)	Husky Cross (1)	Golden Retriever (2)		Rottweiler (2)
	Sheba Inu Shetland Sheepdog Cross (1)	Labrador Retriever (6)	Labrador Retriever (4)		
		Retriever Cross (2)	Labrador Retriever Cross (3)		
		Rottweiler (1)	Mixed Breed (1)		
			Newfoundland (1)		
			Rottweiler (1)		
			Samoyed (2)		

Table 7.2. Characteristics of the dogs pooled from the OCS and CS groups.

Dog Participant Characteristics	
Sex	
Male, Neutered	31 (45.2%)*
Male, Unneutered	2 (4.3%)
Female, Neutered	44 (49.5%)
Female, Unneutered	0 (0%)
Weight, kg	
Mean weight	36.3
Range	7.7 to 45.3
Age, y	
Mean age	5.7
Range	1.1 to 13.0
BCS Categories	
4	4 (5.3%)
5	9 (12.0%)
6	14 (18.7%)
7	25 (33.3%)
8	12 (16.0%)
9	11 (14.7%)

*Values in parentheses indicate the percentage of all participants. Dogs were pooled from the OCS and CS groups.

of the study was significantly correlated with the BCS measured at the end of the assessment period (data not shown). Of further note, the average difference in the number of daily steps per single BCS unit change was $1,935 \pm 478$ steps. This value for the average dog in these studies is almost a kilometer (0.97 km, 0.6 mi) or 10 to 15 minutes of extra walking with a human. This value could prove useful as a very approachable recommendation in a daily exercise program for dogs.

Relative mean body weight of all dogs within each BCS was examined to assure that there were no differences by breed or metabolic energy requirements that may have acted as confounders of the results (Figure 7.4). This effect could potentially skew the results by segregating larger dogs into the higher BCS/lower step categories. Such a contribution may have been present among the BCS category 9 dogs. The mean weight of these dogs was statistically greater

Figure 7.3. Scatter plot of the relationship of average daily step values and baseline BCS. Analysis of these values using Spearman's rank correlation revealed a significant, negative, nonparametric correlation (Spearman's rho=-0.442, p value <0.0001).

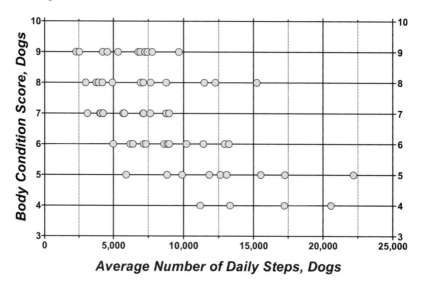

Figure 7.4. Box and whiskers plot of the relationship of body weight and baseline BCS. The upper and lower sides of the boxed area represent the 25th and 75th quartiles of the data. The + mark represents the mean value and the line across the boxed area represents the median. The whiskers represent the range of the maximum and minimum values observed.

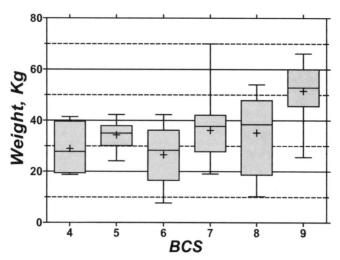

(p-value ≤ 0.01) than all of the other BCS categories; the mean weight of dogs in the other BCS categories did not differ from each other.

There are two potential explanations for the effect seen with the BCS 9 dogs. It could be related to an overall increase in body size of dogs, or this effect could result from an increase in body fat mass. However, there are several reasons why neither of these explanations is likely. First, as is shown in Table 7.1, there was no strong association of any specific breed type with higher or lower BCS values. Second, no change in correlation was seen if these data were adjusted based on relative body fat mass to BCS (Mawby, Bartges, d'Avignon, Laflamme, Moyers, & Cottrell, 2004). This adjustment is based on recent studies measuring fat mass at each BCS using dual-energy X-ray absorptiometry. They reported that an increase in BCS of 1 unit is roughly equal to a 5% increase in fat mass. Further, following adjustment of our results using this value, there was no significant change in the Spearman's correlate suggesting that each nominal increase in BCS is probably not related to fat mass differentials of enrolled dogs (data not shown). Third, it is unlikely that large breed specific inherent basal metabolic rate differences and associated body condition predispositions are playing a prominent role at the higher BCS values. There is limited information regarding breed differences in metabolism with a majority of information being in beagles, Great Danes, Labradors, and Newfoundlands (National Research Council, 2006). While unlikely, if this effect is breed specific, these breeds were not over-represented in our cohorts, and an effect is only seen at the extreme of BCS, a value of 9. As a final argument, our study design did not allow the incorporation of dogs under 10 kg into the study due to the lack of pedometer validity for smaller animals. This further increases the likelihood that each BCS cohort had more similar metabolic rate distribution as potentially higher metabolic rate dogs (small dogs) were not included. More study will be required to resolve this issue.

It can also be argued that this approach may be largely examining the two different subpopulations' feeding practices. Yet when both groups of owners were questioned as to how they fed, across both groups, there were very few owners that actually knew the true quantity of food that was fed, its caloric content, or even the brand of dog food they were using on a daily basis. Knowledge of these three key variables was actually worse in the CS participants. Many of the OCS participants were aware that their dog had a weight problem and were more cognizant of amounts and brands fed. Data were collected from the CS participants for the analysis of energy intake. However, this analysis could not be completed due to poor response rate and clear inaccuracy of reporting. This was disappointing but not surprising. Other studies have found that even when provided detailed questionnaires that correlated well to seven-day dog diet histories, the accuracy of reporting for nutrients or calories has a correlation between 53% and 81% (Laflamme, Kuhlman, & Lawler, 1997).

The major limitation of this study is its observational nature, which does not permit causal discrimination. In addition, the association between BCS and average daily step number presents but does not allow a direct address of the vital question: does a lack of physical activity lead to obesity, or does obesity lead to less physical activity? Walking steps results among the CS owners provide some support for the first of these two possibilities. In this group no difference was observed between the average numbers of daily steps for the owners with normal, overweight, or obese body mass index values (data not shown). Unfortunately, dog owners in the obesity clinic sample cannot be examined in the same manner as they were not asked to report their height and weight or wear pedometers during the study.

Results and discussion, study 3: Dog walking by human participants

Humans involved in the CS arm of the above described studies were also fitted with and trained on the use of pedometers. They were recruited by several avenues: a press release/reporter interview in the local newspaper; a report on a local radio show; and through fliers posted in the local hospital, Humane Society, and Cooperative Extension offices. Participants were provided with paper step logs as well as access to an online step log to post both theirs and their dogs' step counts. Since these studies were carried out as part of the CS dog studies, they followed the same schedule and timeline. That is, the participants were instructed to not change their walking behavior, studies occurred over a 10-week period from early March to mid-May of 2009, and step counts were collected on the first, sixth and tenth weeks of the study. Unlike the dogs, where durability of the pedometers could be an issue, the owners were instructed to wear their pedometers during all their waking hours.

The demographics of the participants are shown in Table 7.3. Participants were largely female, white, and college educated. The mean age was early fifties and almost half of the participants had normal weight range BMI values. Retention of participants for this part of these studies was very good as 90% of these participants completed the study.

In order to place these results into context, the results of this part of the studies are compared to a frequently referenced study in adult humans (Tudor-Locke, Ham, Macera, Ainsworth, Kirtland, Reis, & Kimsey, 2004).

Table 7.3. Characteristics of the recruited human dog walkers from the CS group.

Human Participant Characteristics	
Sex	
Female	36 (75%)*
Male	12 (25%)
Race	
White	47 (98%)
Asian	1 (2%)
Age	
Mean	52
Education	
High School (HS) Graduate	2 (4.2%)
Higher than HS Degree	41 (85.4%
BMI Category	
Underweight	2 (4.4%)
Normal Weight	20 (44.4%)
Overweight	14 (31.1%)
Obese	9 (20%)

*Values in parentheses indicate the percentage of all participants. Differences in total numbers are reflective of voluntary reporting of some characteristics. Participants were from the CS group.

This study was comparable in that it was carried out in a small community, the participants were all adults, and the participants wore pedometers during all waking hours. It differed in that participants were telephone recruited, some of the demographics differed (noted below), and steps were tracked for only one week.

About two thirds of the U.S. population is currently considered overweight or obese. While the population examined in the Tudor-Locke study had overweight/obesity percentages at this level (65%), the recruited population of dog walkers had a lower overall level (54%). The complete BMI distributions of these two populations are shown in Figure 7.5.

Using reported values, the average number of daily steps taken by the dog walkers over three measured weeks was calculated. The overall average was found to be 11,906 steps daily. Average daily step level zones have been described and classified; this daily step level is classified as active (Tudor-Locke, Hatano, Pangrazi, & Kang, 2008). In contrast, the average daily step value from the reference study was one-half the value observed for the dog walking participants, 5,931 steps; this step level is classified as low active. The considerable step difference between what are considered typical U.S. adults and the dog walkers is encouraging. It is important to realize that dog walking participants recruited by local advertizing are far from a random sample

Figure 7.5. Percentage distribution of normal, overweight, and obese human participants in the CS dog walker and reference groups (Tudor-Locke et al., 2004). Values at the base of each column indicate the number of participants in each category for both this figure and for Figure 7.6 (reporting body weight and height was requested but not required).

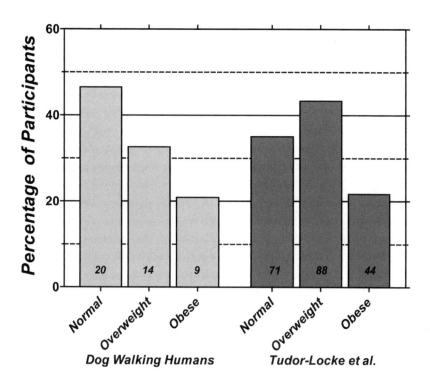

or could even be considered representative of typical dog owners. Nonetheless, the fact that such a considerable step difference exists—even with those that would be considered the most enthusiastic—shows promise for this approach.

Several studies, including the reference walking study, have demonstrated that overweight and obese individuals typically walk less than normal weight individuals (Clemes, Griffiths, & Hamilton, 2007; Clemes, Hamilton, & Lindley, 2008; Tudor-Locke et al., 2001; Tudor-Locke et al., 2004). This pattern is reflected by the bar chart on the right side of Figure 7.6, which represents the average step values for normal, overweight, and obese participants in the reference study. The recruited dog walkers were also exceptional within this context. The average daily step number for the normal and obese dog walkers was surprisingly close to the same values. Obese BMI dog walkers averaged 11,623 steps daily while the average value for dog walkers in the normal BMI range was only 4.5% greater, 12,146 steps.

While the owners of the OCS dogs did not track their walking steps, participants from both owner groups did complete questionnaires that included questions regarding the frequency and duration of walking. The differences in reported dog walking were substantial. While only 25% of the OCS participants agreed that they walked their dog at least once a day, 70% of the CS

Figure 7.6. Average daily step values for the normal, overweight, and obese participants in the CS dog walker and reference groups (Tudor-Locke et al., 2004). Error bars indicate SEM.

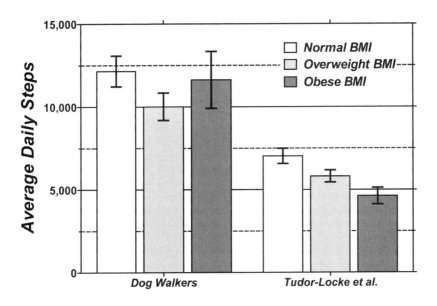

walkers agreed with this statement. Duration of daily walks also differed considerably. Merely 25% of OCS owners agreed that their walks were at least 30 minutes. In contrast, 60% of the CS participants agreed that their walks were at least 30 minutes. Nonetheless, there was no attitudinal difference seen in the importance of the dogs within the family.

Several studies, including unpublished data from our laboratory, have shown that people walk less on weekends (Clemes et al., 2007; Clemes et al., 2008). In contrast, the dog walking group in these studies actually had comparable step values on weekends relative to weekdays (11,860 and 12,063 steps, respectively). Friday step values were consistently high, and the inclusion of Friday with the weekend values produced an increase in the step average that was significant, 12,541 average daily steps from Friday to Sunday versus 10,994 steps from Monday to Thursday (p-value=0.0001). These results further support the potential for dog walking to increase physical activity. The most likely explanation for the increased walking on weekends is that the recruited dog walkers view walking with their dogs as a recreational activity that can be done for longer periods during the free time provided by weekends.

Conclusions

An accurate method for measuring walking steps in medium and large sized dogs was developed. Using this methodology a statistically significant negative correlation was found such that dogs that walked more steps had more favorable BCS. The approximate number of steps between each of the BCS levels was 1,935 steps, which is equivalent to 10 to 15 minutes of extra walking. This added amount of walking on a daily basis might allow a staged approach for dog owners to reduce weight in their dogs. In addition, the step values at each BCS also provide values for daily exercise recommendations. Hence, recommendation to walk approximately 5 to 8 km (3 to 5 mi) or about one hour every day could play a part of a healthful regimen for our canine companions. It is expected that the use of pedometers in dogs will be mostly confined to research environments. Nonetheless, they could have some value for use in dog walking programs or to encourage walking for a canine weight loss program.

The recruited participants most likely better represent an enthusiastic group of dog walkers than the typical dog owner. Nonetheless, the observed results show considerable promise for this approach to increase regular human and canine physical activity. The dog walkers had an overall daily average of 11,906 steps. In contrast, what is considered a typical step level was one half of this value, 5,931 steps (Tudor-Locke et al., 2004). It was also encouraging that the obese dog walkers, in contrast to obese people in general, had a daily average, which was almost that of the normal BMI walkers. Further, this level of walking was 2.5 fold higher than that reported for the obese walkers in the reference study (Clemes et al.,2007; Clemes et al., 2008; Tudor-Locke et al., 2001; Tudor-Locke et al., 2004). These results support the idea that dog walking encourages more daily walking activity. This is certainly a point that needs to be examined in more detail using a group that more closely mirrors the dog owning population. In summation, dog walking is an activity that has great potential to encourage physical activity in both dogs and humans, providing both species with multiple benefits.

Notes

1. Data from the paper or Web-based step logs as well as the owner questionnaires were loaded, managed, and cleaned using standard worksheet software. Analyses were accomplished using STATA or GraphPad Prism software. All data are expressed as means $\pm$ SEM unless otherwise indicated. Basic descriptive statistics, t-tests, and Spearman's correlation analyses were utilized as appropriate to the analysis. A p-value of 0.05 was used for tests of significance.

2. These studies used a 9-point BCS measure of body condition; a BCS of 1 is considered extreme thinness, a BCS of 9 is extreme obesity, and a BCS of 4 or 5 is ideal (Nestlé-Purina, Understanding your dog's body condition. available from http://www.purina.com/dogs/health/bodycondition.aspx).

References

Brener, N. D., Kann, L., Garcia, D., MacDonald, G., Ramsey, F., Honeycutt, S., Hawkins, J. Kinchens, S., & Harris, W. A. (2007). Youth risk behavior surveillance—selected steps communities, 2005. *MMWR Surveillance Summaries, 56*(2), 1-16.

Chan, C. B., Spierenburg, M., Ihle, S. L., & Tudor-Locke, C. (2005). Use of pedometers to measure physical activity in dogs. *Journal of the American Veterinary Medical Association, 226*(12), 2010-2015.

Clemes, S. A., Griffiths, P. L., & Hamilton, S. L. (2007). Four-week pedometer-determined activity patterns in normal weight and overweight UK adults. *International Journal of Obesity (London), 31*(2), 261-266.

Clemes, S. A., Hamilton, S. L., & Lindley, M. R. (2008). Four-week pedometer-determined activity patterns in normal-weight, overweight and obese adults. *American Journal of Preventive Medicine, 46*(4), 325-330.

Corder, K., Brage, S., & Ekelund, U. (2007). Accelerometers and pedometers: Methodology and clinical application. *Current Opinion in Clinical Nutrition & Metabolic Care, 10*(5), 597-603.

Flegal, K. M., Carroll, M. D., Ogden, C. L., & Curtin, L. R. (2010). Prevalence and trends in obesity among US adults, 1999-2008. *Journal of the American Medical Association, 303*(3), 235-241.

German, A. J. (2006). The growing problem of obesity in dogs and cats. *The Journal of Nutrition, 136*(7 Suppl), 1940S-1946S.

Hill, J., Wyatt, H., Reed, G., & Peters, J. (2003). Obesity and the environment: Where do we go from here? *Science, 299*, 853-855.

Hill, J. O., Peters, J. C., & Wyatt, H. R. (2009). Using the energy gap to address obesity: A commentary. *Journal of the American Dietetic Association, 109*(11), 1848-1853.

Hocking, P. M., Bernard, R., & Maxwell, M. H. (1999). Assessment of pain during locomotion and the welfare of adult male turkeys with destructive cartilage loss of the hip joint. *British Poultry Science, 40*(1), 30-34.

Holland, J. L., Kronfeld, D. S., & Meacham, T. N. (1996). Behavior of horses is affected by soy lecithin and corn oil in the diet. *Journal of Animal Science, 74*(6), 1252-1255.

Kruger, J., Ham, S. A., & Kohl, H. W. (2005). Trends in leisure time physical inactivity by age, sex, and race/ethnicity—United States, 1994-2004. *MMWR Surveillance Summaries, 54*(39), 991-994.

Laflamme, D. P. (2006). Understanding and managing obesity in dogs and cats. *Veterinary Clinics of North America: Small Animal Practice, 36*(6), 1283-1295, vii.

Laflamme, D. P., Kuhlman, G., & Lawler, D. F. (1997). Evaluation of weight loss protocols for dogs. *Journal of the American Animal Hospital Association, 33*(3), 253-259.

Mawby, D. I., Bartges, J. W., d'Avignon, A., Laflamme, D. P., Moyers, T. D., & Cottrell, T. (2004). Comparison of various methods for estimating body fat in dogs. *Journal of the American Animal Hospital Association, 40*(2), 109-114.

Mazrier, H., Tal, S., Aizinbud, E., & Bargai, U. (2006). A field investigation of the use of the pedometer for the early detection of lameness in cattle. *Canadian Veterinary Journal, 47*(9), 883-886.

National Research Council. (2006). Energy. In B. C. Beitz (Ed.), *Nutrient requirements of dogs and cats* (pp. 28-48). Washington, DC: National Academy Press.

Ogden, C. L., Yanovski, S. Z., Carroll, M. D., & Flegal, K. M. (2007). The epidemiology of obesity. *Gastroenterology*, *132*(6), 2087-2102.

Roelofs, J. B., van Eerdenburg, F. J., Soede, N. M., & Kemp, B. (2005). Pedometer readings for estrous detection and as predictor for time of ovulation in dairy cattle. *Theriogenology*, *64*(8), 1690-1703.

Sapkota, S., Bowles, H. R., Ham, S. A., & Kohl, H. W. (2005). Adult participation in recommended levels of physical activity—United States, 2001 and 2003. *MMWR Surveillance Summaries*, *54*(47), 1208-1212.

Swinburn, B. A., Sacks, G., Lo, S. K., Westerterp, K. R., Rush, E. C., Rosenbaum, M., Luke, A., Schoeller, D. A., DeLany, J. P., Butte, N. F., Ravussin, E. (2009). Estimating the changes in energy flux that characterize the rise in obesity prevalence. *The Journal of Nutrition*, *89*(6), 1723-1728.

Tudor-Locke, C., Ainsworth, B. E., Whitt, M. C., Thompson, R. W., Addy, C. L., & Jones, D. A. (2001). The relationship between pedometer-determined ambulatory activity and body composition variables. *International Journal of Obesity*, *25*(11), 1571-1578.

Tudor-Locke, C., Ham, S. A., Macera, C. A., Ainsworth, B. E., Kirtland, K. A., Reis, J. P., et al. (2004). Descriptive epidemiology of pedometer-determined physical activity. *Medicine & Science in Sports & Exercise*, *36*(9), 1567-1573.

Tudor-Locke, C., Hatano, Y., Pangrazi, R. P., & Kang, M. (2008). Revisiting "how many steps are enough?" *Medicine & Science in Sports & Exercise*, *40*(7 Suppl), S537-543.

Westerterp, K. R. (1999). Physical activity assessment with accelerometers. *International Journal of Obesity*, *23*(Suppl 3), S45-49.

Yaissle, J. E., Holloway, C., & Buffington, C. A. (2004). Evaluation of owner education as a component of obesity treatment programs for dogs. *Journal of the American Veterinary Medical Association*, *224*(12), 1932-1935.

Chapter 8

Dog obesity, dog walking, and dog health

Karyl J. Hurley, Denise A. Elliott, and Elizabeth Lund

Other chapters in this volume focus on the benefits of dog walking for people; however, clearly there are also shared benefits and risks for dogs. Depending on their size, breed, and temperament, some dogs need more exercise than others to maintain their fitness level, keep them from becoming bored and destructive, and, perhaps most importantly, to provide mental stimulation, socialization, and simply entertainment (Defra, 2009). As reported by Chauvet, exercise can also significantly increase the rate of weight loss in overweight or obese pets (Chauvet, Laclai, Elliott, & German, 2010). However, whether you are walking with a shelter dog or your own pet, benefits will be shared from the activity as long as the health and welfare of the dog are kept front of mind.

Tackling obesity in dogs

Scope and magnitude of overweight and obesity in the dogs

Much attention has been given to the current obesity epidemic in the U.S. human population. It has been estimated that two-thirds of humans in the U.S. are overweight or obese (Flegal, Carroll, Ogden, & Johnson, 2002); the prevalence of obesity alone between 2004-2006 was estimated to be over 33% (Ogden et al., 2006). Overweight or obese humans are at greater risk of type 2 diabetes mellitus, hypertension, coronary artery disease, osteoarthritis, respiratory disease, reproductive disorders, and certain cancers (e.g., breast, ovarian, and prostate) (Avenell et al., 2004; Houston, Nicklas, & Zizza, 2009; Kolonin, Saha, Chan, Pasqualini, & Arap, 2004; Prevention, 2009).

The prevalence of canine obesity has been estimated at between 22.4% and 44% (Hill, 2009; Lund, 1999; McGreevy et al., 2005), and most researchers agree that the prevalence of pet obesity is increasing in a similar fashion to human obesity (German, 2006). Are there pet and owner specific factors that can help us identify which dogs are at greatest risk? These dogs are even more likely to benefit from dog walking.

Risk factors for canine obesity

Many risk factors for overweight and obesity in dogs have been identified, including genetics, concurrent diseases, age, breed, gender, diet, lifestyle, and attributes of the pet-owner bond. Risk factors represent associations that may or may not be causal, but help understand patterns in populations that can elucidate causality.

In dogs, Labrador retrievers, Cairn terriers, Cavalier King Charles spaniels, Scottish terriers, cocker spaniels, dalmatians, dachshunds, rottweilers, golden retrievers, Shetland sheepdogs, and "mixed" breeds have been identified as being at increased risk of being overweight or obese (German, 2006; E. Lund, 2006). The top 10 breeds at greatest risk from the Banfield database[1] (Table 8.1) include: pug, beagle, golden retriever, Labrador retriever, dachshund, dalmatian, Shetland sheepdog, Australian shepherd, rottweiler, and American cocker spaniel (Lund, 2007).

Although data on the effects of overweight or obesity on dogs is more limited than that in humans, research suggests that they may be predisposed to orthopedic disease, diabetes mellitus, abnormalities in circulating lipid profiles, cardiorespiratory disease, urinary disorders, reproductive disorders, dermatological diseases, and neoplasia (e.g., mammary tumors and transitional cell carcinoma) (German, 2006). Concurrent diseases found to be associated with overweight or obesity include endocrine dysfunction (low thyroid hormones [hypothyroidism] and excess adrenal hormones, such as overproduction of steroids [hyperadrenocorticism], infection-related obesity, cruciate ligament rupture, lower urinary tract disease, oral disease, diabetes mellitus, pancreatitis and neoplasia (Laflamme, 2006; Lund, 2006). In the Banfield population, the highest risk for concurrent disease (Table 8.2) was for hypothyroidism, hyperadrenocorticism, diabetes, eyelid margin tumor, and arthritis. These are diseases that were more likely to be diagnosed in dogs that were also overweight or obese at the time of the visit to the veterinarian.

Anesthetic risk has also been reported to be increased in overweight or obese dogs (German, 2006). Overweight or obese dogs have been shown to require medication for osteoarthritis three years earlier than dogs of a normal

Table 8.1. Top ten dogs at risk for overweight/obesity by breed—% breed distribution by body condition.

Breed	Obese Dogs	Non-obese Dogs	Relative Risk*
Pug	2.3%	0.8%	2.8
Beagle	4.4%	2.0%	2.3
Golden retriever	6.3%	3.3%	2.0
Labrador retriever	17.8%	10.9%	1.8
Dachshund	4.4%	2.9%	1.6
Dalmatian	1.5%	1.1%	1.5
Shetland sheepdog	2.2%	1.4%	1.5
Australian shepherd	1.8%	1.3%	1.4
Rottweiler	4.1%	3.4%	1.2
American cocker spaniel	5.5%	4.8%	1.1

*Measure of the association between breed and overweight/obesity.

Table used with permission from Banfield, The Pet Hospital.

weight (Kealy et al., 2000). Overweight or obese humans do not live as long as humans of a healthy body weight (Houston et al., 2009; Kolonin et al., 2004; Prevention, 2009), and there is evidence to suggest that this is also the case in dogs (Kealy et al., 2000). In the latter study, dogs kept lean from puppyhood outlived their littermates who had access to freely available food, and therefore were overweight by two years; the lean dogs lived on average to 14 years, whereas the overweight dogs lived on average to 12 years of age.

Pet-specific factors associated with overweight or obesity include age, gender, neuter status, less than daily exercise, and residential area. Middle-aged, female gender, and sterilized dogs are more likely to be overweight or obese (German, 2006; Kronfeld, Donoghue, & Glickman, 1991; Laflamme, 2006; Lund, 2006; McGreevy et al., 2005). In addition, daily exercise is associated with healthy body weight (Bland et al., 2009). Where a dog resides has also been found to be important; dogs in rural or semi-rural areas were more likely to be overweight or obese than dogs in urban or suburban areas (McGreevy et al., 2005). This is ironic, as a lack of activity is also associated with overweight or obesity in dogs (Laflamme, 2006), and one might anticipate that dogs in rural areas with potential access to larger roaming territories

Table 8.2. Canine prevalence of and risk for concurrent disease by overweight/ obesity status—% disease prevalence by body condition.

	Obese	Non-obese	Relative Risk
Hypothyroidism	3.9%	0.8%	5.3
Hyperadrenocorticism	0.6%	0.1%	5.1
Diabetes	0.7%	0.2%	3.4
Eyelid margin tumor	0.6%	0.2%	3.1
Arthritis	7.1%	2.7%	2.8
Mast cell tumor	0.5%	0.2%	2.7
Oral disease	71.4%	50.2%	2.5
Skin tumors	6.4%	2.9%	2.3
Osteoarthritis	0.8%	0.3%	2.3
Perianal gland tumor	0.1%	.04%	2.2
Ruptured anterior cruciate ligament	1.0%	0.5%	2.0
Pancreatitis	1.2%	0.6%	1.9
Oral neoplasia	0.4%	0.2%	1.9
Urinary disease	6.3%	3.8%	1.7
Respiratory disease	3.9%	2.6%	1.5
Mammary neoplasia	0.3%	0.2%	1.4
Dermatologic disease	45.7%	37.9%	1.4
Constipation	0.34%	0.25%	1.3
Cardiovascular disease	5.2%	4.4%	1.2

Table used with permission from Banfield, The Pet Hospital.

might exercise more and hence be of a healthier weight. Perhaps, dogs that reside in rural areas also have greater access to foods with high caloric density (e.g., table scraps, they may hunt for food, or perhaps spend more time tethered), but this is speculation.

Not surprisingly, high-fat diets are associated with overweight or obesity in dogs (Laflamme, 2006). However, the source of food (commercially prepared vs. homemade) does not appear to predispose to overweight or obesity (Kienzle et al., 1998). The price of the pet food, however, does have an effect; overweight or obese dogs are more likely to be fed inexpensive foods. An association has also been found between the number of meals and snacks fed as well as feeding of kitchen/table scraps, fresh meat, and commercial treats (Bland et al., 2009; Kienzle et al., 1998).

Over-humanization of animals is associated with overweight or obesity in dogs (Kienzle et al., 1998). Owners of overweight or obese dogs often relate to their pets as children or family members and even as substitutes for human companionship. This is evidenced by owners of overweight or obese dogs reportedly speaking to their pets and allowing them to sleep on the bed more often than owners of normal weight pets. They also were less concerned about zoonotic disease and rated exercise, work, or protection by the dog as less important reasons for ownership as compared to owners of dogs of normal weight. These owners perceive food as a convenient and acceptable form of communication and interaction with their pets and spend more time watching their pet eat. These pets were also more likely to be present when the owner prepared or ate their own meals and were fed tidbits at these times.

From this same study population, it was found that an owner's interest in his or her pet's nutrition and his or her own nutrition is related to both the pet and his or her own obesity status (Kienzle et al., 1998). Overweight or obese owners had less interest in their pet's preventive health care than owners of normal weight dogs. However, neither group (normal pet weight or obese) felt that preventive health care was the most important reason to visit the veterinarian (Kienzle et al., 1998). Owners of overweight or obese dogs also had less interest in their own preventive health care and were less interested in providing balanced nutrition for their dog than owners of normal weight dogs.

Human risk factors for pet obesity include exercise habits and owner income (Kienzle et al., 1998; Courcier et. al 2010). Owners of overweight or obese dogs have a lower net income than owners of normal weight dogs and are less likely to participate in regular exercise. In one study, increased owner age was found to be positively associated with increased risk for pet overweight or obesity (Courcier et al., 2010). Despite understanding of the myriad pet and owner factors that influence dog overweight and obesity, it remains a challenge for veterinarians and dog owners.

Another recent study attempting to further understand the complex human-pet interaction and relationship to pet obesity used the theory of planned behavior to explore the connection of owners' beliefs, feeding and exercise intentions, feeding and exercise behaviors, and body condition scores of their pets (Rohlf, Toukhsati, Coleman, & Bennett, 2010). The findings reveal that despite good intentions, pet owners still have overweight pets, and either they are unaware that their pet is obese or they are not significantly motivated to change this condition. This has resounding implications for how we create strategies for pet owners going forward.

Diagnosis of obesity

Prevention of obesity is ideal, but due to poor education, lack of motivation, or understanding of health implications, weight management or weight loss can be a difficult course for many pet owners. The diagnosis of obesity is seemingly straightforward when a pet becomes rather rotund, but it is remarkable how infrequently the diagnosis is either recognized by the owner as a problem or documented in a medical record by the veterinarian. Indeed, underreporting of the diagnosis by veterinarians is routine; Lund et al. (1999) found that although 28% of dogs seen at veterinary practices in the United States were identified as overweight or obese by their body condition scores (BCS), only 2% were actually diagnosed as obese. German found that of 148 dogs examined by veterinarians in the United Kingdom, only 70% had documented a body weight, 29% had a recorded assessment of body condition (e.g., thin, ideal, or obese), and only one had a BCS noted in their patient record (German & Morgan, 2008). Furthermore, it is the authors' collective belief that veterinary education in nutritional sciences, including the cause and prevention of obesity, is sadly lacking in most veterinary training programs. We speculate that this may be due to the commonality of overly crowded curricula focused on the understanding of disease processes with less emphasis on preventive medicine.

Obesity is defined by an excess accumulation of body fat. There are numerous techniques available to assess the degree of body fat, however, only the clinically relevant techniques will be discussed in this chapter. Information on advanced and research techniques including dilutional techniques, bioelectrical impedance analysis, dual energy X-ray absorptiometry, densitometry, computed tomography, magnetic resonance imaging, total body electrical conductivity, total body potassium, and neutron activation analysis can be found in many additional resources.

Body weight is the simplest technique used to assess body composition. It provides a rough measure of total body energy stores and changes in weight parallel energy and protein balance. In the healthy dog, body weight varies little from day to day. There can be wide variation between scales though, so it is important to use the same scale for an individual dog each time to avoid inter-scale variation. In addition, it is preferable to routinely calibrate the scale to maintain accuracy. However, a measurement of body weight by itself has little meaning. Knowing that a Labrador weighs 68 pounds means little; the dog could be overweight, underweight, or in ideal body condition. Therefore, body weight should not be used in isolation. In addition, body weight can be falsely altered in disease by dehydration or fluid accumulation.

BCS provides a quick and subjective assessment of a pet's overall body condition (Laflamme, 1997). The two most commonly used scoring systems in small animal practice are a 5-point system where a BCS of 3 is considered ideal (Figure 8.1). BCS in conjunction with body weight provides a more complete perspective on a pet's body condition and should be recorded by the veterinarian at every visit. Owners can be taught how to use BCS to monitor their dog's weight loss status and/or to maintain a healthy weight. Limitations of BCS include the subjectivity inherent in the scoring system and interobserver variation.

Management of canine obesity

The management of obesity is a complex process that requires the interaction and coordination of the entire veterinary medical team. Obesity management requires an integrated approach to incorporate nutritional recommendations, owner education, and exercise as well as behavioral aspects, such as not feeding table scraps and allowing the pet to reside under the table at meal times. Most importantly to achieve success, the pet owner needs to be completely committed to the program and motivated to comply with the directions.

Owner engagement in the management of the overweight or obese pet is critical. The first step in the process is to make sure that the owner both realizes that their pet is overweight or obese, and equally important, realizes that this is a serious medical condition with a number of life-threatening consequences for the pet, in addition to the economical and emotional consequences for the pet owner. The owners must understand that weight loss will improve the health of their dogs (Roudebush, Schoenherr, & Delaney, 2008). The veterinarian and veterinary team is responsible for making the diagnosis of obesity of the pet, for providing the appropriate client education on the health risks of being overweight or obese, for prescribing the appropriate therapeutic treatment tailored for the individual needs of the pet and the owner, and for ensuing consistent supervision and advice by members of the veterinary health care team. The veterinary health care team should be supportive of the pet and owner at all times, avoid criticism for relapses, and always provide constructive, helpful advice. With the high incidence of overweight and obesity in the human population, some members of the veterinary health care team may be embarrassed to broach the topic of overweight or obesity management with the pet owner. However, the veterinary team is responsible for the health of the pet, and hence the conversation should always be focused on the pet.

Once the owner is ready to implement a treatment plan for his or her

Figure 8.1. Body condition score in dogs. The chart below is a guide to assessing a dog's body condition. Please note that some breeds and different life stages may have different ideal body condition scores. Retrieved from http://www.royalcanin.co.uk/my_pet/puppy_guide/dog_body_condition.aspx

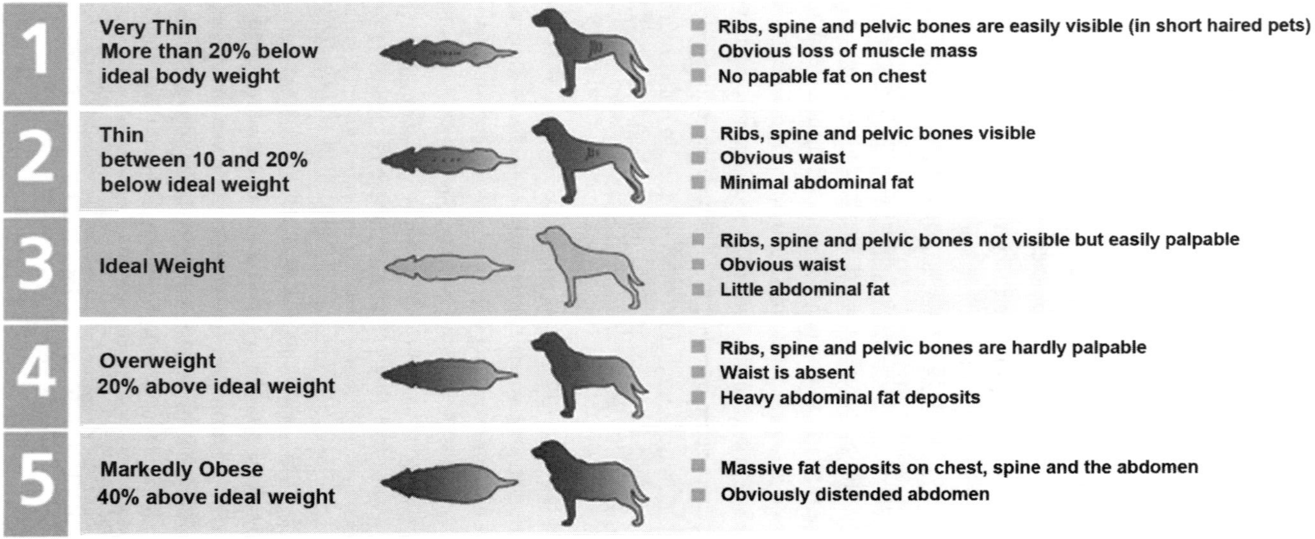

1 Very Thin
More than 20% below ideal body weight
- Ribs, spine and pelvic bones are easily visible (in short haired pets)
- Obvious loss of muscle mass
- No papable fat on chest

2 Thin
between 10 and 20% below ideal weight
- Ribs, spine and pelvic bones visible
- Obvious waist
- Minimal abdominal fat

3 Ideal Weight
- Ribs, spine and pelvic bones not visible but easily palpable
- Obvious waist
- Little abdominal fat

4 Overweight
20% above ideal weight
- Ribs, spine and pelvic bones are hardly palpable
- Waist is absent
- Heavy abdominal fat deposits

5 Markedly Obese
40% above ideal weight
- Massive fat deposits on chest, spine and the abdomen
- Obviously distended abdomen

overweight or obese dog, a thorough dietary history should be obtained. Information that should be gathered includes:

- The name, manufacturer, and type (i.e., canned versus dry) of the current diet

- The amount of diet that is fed each day (can versus cups of food; always verify the size of the cup the owner is using)

- The energy provided within the diet fed—kilocalories per cup or can

- The method of feeding (food freely available versus meal fed)

- The person responsible for feeding the dog

- Additional persons that may feed the dog (especially children, elderly parents, or friendly neighbors)

- The number and type of snacks or human foods given each day

- Access to other pets' food

This dietary information should be used to calculate the daily caloric intake of the dog. The dog's current body weight should be recorded, and the target body weight of the dog should be calculated. The ideal body weight can be estimated by referring to breed body weight charts. Alternatively, and perhaps more appropriate for each individual, is to review the body weight history of the pet over his or her lifespan. Typically, the body weight of the dog as a young adult most closely approximates the ideal body weight.

The amount of calories to feed the dog is determined on the basis of the target body weight. Several equations exist to calculate the number of calories required for weight loss. The authors typically recommend feeding 50% to 60% of the maintenance requirements for ideal body weight: $0.45 \times (132 \times \text{Ideal Body Weight kg}^{0.73})$ (Table 8.3). The amount of calories required for weight loss should be compared to the actual daily intake. In rare situations, the amount of calories to achieve weight loss is actually less than the current daily caloric intake. Therefore, before beginning the weight loss plan, the dietary history should be reevaluated to search for additional calories. If no additional daily calories are identified, then the daily caloric intake of the dog for ideal body weight should be reduced by 15%.

Once the daily caloric requirement to achieve ideal body weight has been calculated, consideration should be given to the type of diet to feed. There are essentially two main dietary options to be considered, either feed a reduced amount of the regular maintenance diet, or feed a diet that has been specifically formulated for weight reduction. Often the pet owner wants to feed less of the current diet, however, this is not advisable as this was the diet

Table 8.3. Example of how to calculate the energy requirements for weight loss in overweight or obese dogs.

As an example, you have a six-year-old female spay mixed breed dog who currently weighs 52 pounds. She has a body condition score of 4/5. You estimate her ideal body weight should be 44 pounds. Caloric intake for weight loss=0.45 x (132 x ideal BW $kg^{0.73}$). Note, you need to convert the current body weight data from lbs to kg. 1 lb=0.45359237 kg. Therefore, the number of calories per day for this dog=0.45 x (132 x (44 x 0.45359237)$^{0.73}$

= 0.45 x (132 x (19.96)$^{0.73}$)

= 0.45 x (132 x 8.89)

= 0.45 x 1174

= 528 kcal per day for weight loss.

that led to the problem in the first place, and old habits are hard to change. More importantly, feeding a maintenance diet increases the risk of nutrient deficiency and unhealthy weight loss. Canine maintenance diets are formulated according to energy intake. This means that if a dog eats its daily energy requirement, it will automatically consume the required amounts of additional essential nutrients such as amino acids, vitamins, and minerals. By feeding less of the maintenance diet, you are not only reducing the amount of energy, but also are reducing the amount of protein, essential fatty acids, vitamins, and minerals, and thereby may risk malnutrition. Conversely, diets that have been specifically formulated for weight reduction contain more essential nutrients relative to the energy content of the diet. This means that the dog will receive the required amounts of proteins, vitamins, and minerals, even though they are ingesting less energy.

Diets formulated specifically for weight reduction will vary predominantly according to the fiber, protein, and energy content. High fiber diets have been suggested for weight loss because certain types of fiber provide a satiating effect (Jewell & Toll, 1996). High dietary fiber content will reduce the digestibility of the diet, and increases the amount of fecal material, which can be burdensome in large and giant breed dogs, or for pets in apartment dwelling situations. High protein diets have been reported to increase the proportion of fat loss while preserving or indeed increasing the lean body mass (Diez et al., 2002). The lean body mass is the most metabolically active portion of the body and includes skeletal muscle tissues. Preservation of lean body mass has been shown to facilitate successful long-term maintenance of ideal body weight once weight loss has been achieved. The effect of energy restricted diets containing a macronutrient combination that is both high in fiber and high in protein have also been reported to be effective in the management of weight loss in dogs (German, Holden, Bissot, Morris, & Biourge; Weber et al., 2007).

The energy content of diets designed for weight loss can also vary rather dramatically (Linder & Freeman, 2010). By example, Linder et al. reported that canine dry diets with weight management claims range from 217 to 440 kilocalories per cup, and feline dry diets vary from 235 to 480 kilocalories per cup (Linder & Freeman, 2010). Although it is impossible to understand the rationale behind these differences, these variations could reflect differences between manufactures that are purely marketing driven, versus those that have the expertise and knowledge to formulate the diets on the nutritional needs of the pet. It is important when considering diets to determine if they are actually designed for weight loss, and are hence calorically restricted, or if they are actually designed for weight maintenance of dogs predisposed to weight gain. These "light" diets may indeed contain fewer calories than all other products within a particular brand's range of foods but in reality are not as energy restricted as those diets that are specifically designed for therapeutic weight loss. An additional consideration is the energy density of the diet, that is, how many kilocalories of diet per cup or per can of food. A good weight loss diet will contain fewer calories per cup or can. Lowering the energy density of food actually allows a reasonable volume of food to be provided to the pet, and will therefore lessen the likelihood of the owner feeling guilty by the extreme volume restriction. Consider the following example: an eight-year-old male neutered Labrador who currently weighs 47 kg. His estimated ideal body weight should be 35 kg. His caloric requirement for weight loss is approximately 796 kcal per day. One diet specifically designed for weight loss contains 235 kcal per cup compared with an alternative weight loss diet that contains 325 kcal per cup. The difference between the amounts fed each day for the two diets translates to 3.4 cups versus 2.4 cups. This is a clinically relevant difference for both the owner and the pet's perception.

Carnitine is an additional nutrient that is vital for energy metabolism and can be considered in weight loss diets. Carnitine facilitates the movement of long chain fatty acids across the mitochondrial membrane where the long chain fatty acids can be used for energy production. Carnitine supplementation may facilitate fat loss and maintain lean body mass.

Ideally, the dog should be meal fed rather than having food freely available at all times. The number of feedings per day can be selected to suit the owners' schedule, but two to four meals per day are adequate. One member of the household should be selected to feed the dog. This will reduce inadvertent over feeding by additional family members. The actual size of the cup should also be verified with the owner. Feeding guides in North America are developed on the basis of a standard U.S. cup, which is 8 ounces or 237 milliliters. Correctly sized measuring cups can be readily and inexpensively obtained at home goods stores or are often provided by pet food manufacturers. Kitchen scales provide an even more accurate method of weighing the correct amount of food to offer each day.

The owner should eliminate treats completely, or if this is met with resistance, treats should be limited to less than 10% of the daily caloric intake. Ideally, low calorie treats should be selected. Ice-cubes, carrots, or other vegetables make effective low calorie treats, especially for large breed dogs. It is also worthwhile exploring why and when the dog receives treats. In many instances, treats are used inappropriately to appease owner guilt (e.g., arriving home late, leaving early), rather than as a reward. In these situations, owner behavior of feeding treats can be readily replaced by additional objects of affection such as games, toys, and petting.

Additional owner behaviors should be modified (e.g., not allowing the dog into the kitchen or dining room during meal preparation or consumption). This will reduce the likeliness of the owner giving the dog human snacks, which are generally high in calories. In addition, the owner should inform and enlist the support of other family members and neighbors in the weight reduction program so that they do not unknowingly give the dog additional calories. In some cases, it may be useful to utilize a food diary to record the amount of food and snacks fed each day. Food diaries are particularly useful to understand difficulties achieving weight loss.

Various pharmaceutical agents have been evaluated for treatment of obesity in dogs, cats, and humans. Dirlotapide, (Slentrol®, Pfizer) a microsomal triglyceride transfer protein inhibitor, has been developed specifically for weight reduction in dogs and has been shown to be effective; however, rebound weight gain occurs at the end of treatment when appropriate diet and exercise strategies are not in place (Gossellin, McKelvie, et al., 2007; Gossellin, Peachey, Sherington, Rowan, & Sunderland, 2007; Wren et al., 2007). Successful weight management plans require diagnosis and awareness of the significance of the condition by the veterinary team and the owner, agreement and commitment to the weight management plan, the appropriate dietary regimen, exercise, and behavioral modification.

Dogs on weight reduction programs should be reevaluated every two to four weeks. Body weight and BCS should be recorded. The dietary history should be reviewed. Typically, with pets in the home environment, the average rate of weight loss is 0.8% per week (German, Holden, Bissot, Hackett, & Biourge, 2007). If the body weight loss is less than 1%, then the daily caloric intake should be reduced by 10% to 15%. Conversely, if the rate of weight loss exceeds 3% body weight loss per week, the daily caloric intake should be increased by 10% to 15%.

Exercise should be used in combination with dietary management to promote fat loss and assist in lean tissue preservation. In dogs, suitable exercise strategies include leash walking (see below), swimming, hydrotherapy, and treadmills. Chauvet et al. reported in a case-control pilot study that exercise in combination with a traditional weight loss and education program was associated with a significant increase in the rate of weight loss per week in client-owned overweight and obese pets (Chauvet, Laclai, Elliott, & German, 2010). Further studies are necessary to refine the best recommendations for incorporating exercise into weight management programs.

Prevention of obesity

The key to preventing obesity is owner education. Energy requirements decrease when the dog is sterilized. Therefore, active steps toward obesity prevention should begin at the time of neutering. Owners should be taught the risk factors (age, sex, breed, life-style, inappropriate feeding practices) and consequences of obesity. Importantly, owners should be instructed on how to feed their dog, how to regularly determine body condition, and how to adjust the amount that they feed their dog to maintain ideal body condition. The significance of exercise in helping to maintain healthy body weight should be reinforced. These critical health recommendations should be reinforced at each annual or biennial health examination.

Dog walking: Beyond obesity—addressing the welfare of the dog

Just as dog walking has beneficial effects for people, dog walking can have equally important beneficial health effects for dogs, especially in the treatment and management of overweight or obesity. However, it is essential to ensure that the welfare of the dog is addressed. This includes dog-human walking compatibility, ensuring that the dog is healthy and fit, providing for its safety from environmental dangers, and monitoring hydration and physical status.

Dog-human walking compatibility

Dog-human walking compatibility will facilitate success and mutual benefit for both ends of the leash. First, is the dog's health and fitness up to walking the desired distances? All dogs should be in good muscle condition, have routine annual veterinary preventative care, and current vaccinations prior to potential exposure to other dogs and people. Dogs of all breeds and sizes may enjoy being walked, however, their individual fitness levels, temperaments, and predisposition to exercise must be taken into account. The same holds true for the humans, so there needs to be a match between the dog and human energy levels, strength, and enthusiasm. All dog walking partners should have had some behavioral training; they should be able to walk on a leash without pulling and follow simple commands such as "sit" and "stay." They must be of good temperament with people and with other animals. Dogs should show interest in dog-dog and dog-human interaction and exhibit friendly, non-threatening behaviors like sniffing and tail wagging. Dogs with aggressive tendencies should not be walked in areas where there is a high potential for interaction with people, dogs, or other animals. They must be kept under tight leash control at all times and preferably should be wearing a soft cloth muzzle or training harness.

Puppies over 16 weeks may be walked as part of their socialization program, but not for long distances since their bones and joints are still developing. Dogs can handle extended walks as they reach adulthood at 9 to 12 months for small breeds and 15 months for large breeds. Larger dogs may have greater endurance and exercise tolerance than smaller dogs, and so they can likely manage longer and faster paced jaunts. Younger dogs may have higher energy levels than older animals, and neutered dogs are less likely to be distracted by sights and smells of other dogs than intact males. These latter observations are of course generalizations, recognizing that dogs are individuals with differing personalities and preferences. Dogs with diagnosed health issues may still be exercised on walks, but depending upon the specific problem, extra care must be taken not to exacerbate the condition, and knowledge of the nearest veterinary practice is always a good piece of information to have on hand. For dogs with orthopedic issues—arthritis, stiff joints, or tendons—long distance walking is probably not a good option, but short walks at a leisurely pace may be beneficial to keep their joints mobile and flexible. Prophylactic non-steroidal anti-inflammatory drugs may be prescribed by a veterinarian to ameliorate the pain associated with arthritis, and if post-exercise pain is evident, the dog should no longer participate until the condition improves. For more severely affected dogs, swimming may be an activity better suited to supporting their limbs while they are active, so as to not overstress or further damage joints and tendons.

Overweight and obese dogs have greater stress on their joints, and pressure on their thoracic cavity from intra-abdominal fat accumulation, so they may not have the endurance of a dog of normal weight. They are also more prone to heat stress, so although the long-term benefits of exercise and weight loss may be realized, walks should be perhaps slower, shorter, and incrementally increased as part of a calorie-restricted diet and exercise program under the guidance of a veterinarian. Unlike in people, there is no prescribed "30 minutes a day" time for exercise. This must be tailored to the energy levels of the dog and the owner. Dogs with clinical respiratory disease, overt pain, or lameness should not be walked.

Dog walking equipment—the essentials

Basic dog walking equipment includes a collar or harness, a leash, water, and potentially toys. The collar should be snug-fitting so the dog is not able to slip out of it, yet loose enough to allow for comfort. A harness may be better suited for small breeds whereby no pressure is placed on the trachea, which can exacerbate tracheal collapse common to small breed dogs. The leash may be a retractable or fixed-length lead. The retractable leads are often less preferred by some behaviorists as the fixed lead is of constant predictable length and affords better control of the dog (Westgarth et al., 2009). Access to water is important, and ideally, either a fresh water source is available during the walk or water is brought along in a thermos with a bowl or collapsible cup for frequent hydration stops. Exercise caution when allowing dogs to drink from ponds or streams, as infectious organisms such as *Giardia* and *Leptospirosis* may be transmitted through stagnant pools of water where deer or cattle have had access (Greene, 2006).

There are many varied types of toys on the market that can make a walk more fun for the dog and the owner/handler (e.g., www.activedogtoys.com/outdoor) provided there is safe space to let the dog off the leash to pursue Frisbees, balls, or other water impermeable, easily washable items of play. This is an especially effective form of exercise for highly energetic or exuberant dogs that perhaps need to expend more energy than the handler can manage.

Finally, all dogs should have some form of identification, such as a name tag with a phone number on the collar at the very least. Some areas of the U.S. require a rabies vaccination tag on the collar as well. Ideally, all pets should have an embedded microchip that can be read by a shelter or veterinarian to identify the owner should a dog go astray or get lost.

Where to walk a dog

Trails, sidewalks, dog parks, cities, neighborhoods, countryside, beaches—where one can legally walk a dog depends on what is available to one wherever he or she may live or travel. Certain areas have restrictions on where one can walk dogs, so awareness of any regulations about leashes and pet accessibility is crucial. The environment can pose a number of challenges one must recognize when dog walking, such as foreign materials, like a piece of glass that may be ingested or stepped on causing injury. Interactions with other dogs, vehicles, wildlife, people, and infectious agents all pose potential threats to the dogs' health and welfare if not appropriately recognized and minimized where possible.

Regardless of where one walks his or her dog, it should be safe from oncoming traffic (e.g., off the road onto a sidewalk or trail). There should be suitable terrain for soft footpads such as grass, sand, or dirt paths. Avoid hot pavement, rough coral, littered glass, or thorny "off-the-beaten–paths" that can cause footpad injuries. A plastic bag or poop-scoop should always be accessible for use in removing feces from public places. Dog parks, where dogs are allowed off-leash to freely roam and play with other visiting dogs and owners in an open yet confined space, are becoming increasingly popular (www.dog-park.com). Although the dog handlers may not get as much exercise as they would walking alongside the dog, an added mutual benefit is the opportunity to interact socially with other pets, pet owners, and park users, expanding or enhancing social networks and improving pet socialization skills (www.healthyparkshealthypeople.com).

When to walk a dog

There is no ideal time of day or year to walk a dog, but there are a few important considerations regarding seasonal temperatures and weather conditions. In hot weather, heat exhaustion can easily overcome dogs of any size or shape. There are physical characteristics of breeds that may predispose them to heat exhaustion and therefore warrant extra caution when exercising in warm weather. Dogs with thick fur coats, such as huskies or Samoyeds may succumb to heat exhaustion more readily, as well as dogs with dark fur that more easily absorbs and holds heat longer than lighter colored dogs. Brachycephalic breeds, such as bulldogs and Boston terriers, have excessive pharyngeal tissue and more narrow respiratory passages than dolichocephalic dogs (such as German shepherds) and therefore cannot readily pant to cool themselves like other breeds. Finally, dogs do not sweat, which does not allow the skin to cool down by evaporation as occurs in humans.

Heat tolerance and stamina is lower in obese dogs compared with those of normal weight (Lund, 2007). The most common early clinical signs of heat exhaustion are excessive panting, leading to weakness, loss of balance, excessive salivation, and if left untreated, heat exhaustion can progress to mental dullness, collapse, and even death (Mazzafero, 2010). Whenever an animal appears to be overheated, stop all activity, find a shady spot to rest, and provide water. If there is a source of cool water, such as a stream or faucet, douse the dog with water and apply cold water or ice to the footpads. If the signs do not fully resolve within minutes, then the dog should be taken to an emergency veterinarian. Immediate treatment is critical to success when dealing with heat exhaustion, and delays are potentially harmful or fatal.

To prevent issues with overheating, avoid walking dogs in the heat of the day and direct sunlight. Instead, an early morning walk, an excursion at dusk, or staying within areas where there is plenty of shade are better choices. Know the warning signs and be sensitive to the dog's needs; take frequent breaks for water; take a shorter route or stop altogether if the dog is panting incessantly and slows down. Hydration can be assessed by lifting the lip and checking that the gums are pink and wet, and when pressed with a finger, quickly turn from white to pink again (capillary refill time). If the gums are red, dry, and slow to refill, the dog should be taken for veterinary care.

In colder weather, dogs can suffer damage to their footpads after being exposed to cold, icy surfaces during the winter months. Limit time outdoors when icy conditions prevail, and take special care that your dog does not drink from puddles in urban areas, as they could be contaminated with ethylene glycol, a common component of antifreeze that is toxic for dogs. Small or short-haired breed dogs may benefit from a dog sweater for extended outdoor activities.

Managing interactions

On occasion, dogs will be distracted from walking by other dogs, people, wildlife, and nearly any object that has a scent. A dog's sense of smell is said to be a thousand times more sensitive than that of humans, and their olfactory sense is an effective form of communication when they mark their territories with urine or lead with their nose to inspect new objects, people, and dogs. To decrease the possibility of negative interactions, dogs should be kept under control on a leash when in public places (Westgarth et al., 2009). Dog-dog or dog-person encounters can be avoided by keeping the dog leashed close to your side until the dog or person passes. A short leash can be very useful in avoiding antagonistic encounters as long as both dogs are appropriately managed on a leash (Bradshaw & Lea, 1992). If an encounter does occur, it usually involves mutual sniffing and inspection among well socialized dogs. However, be alert to any potential aggression and be prepared to pull the leash back in order to separate the dogs safely. Since a dog's olfactory inspections concentrate on the head and anal regions, respiratory and gastrointestinal infectious agents can be transmitted from dog to dog, or from a contaminated environment to dogs (Westgarth, 2010). Bacterial and viral agents that are possible to be passed on from such encounters may include *Bordetella* (kennel cough), parvovirus, coronavirus, *Campylobacter*, and even rabies. However, serious pathogens are less likely to be encountered as known carriers or ill animals should be isolated rather than allowed to be outside with potential for exposing other pets. Preventing dogs from inspecting, ingesting, or rolling in feces or alternative food sources along the route will also minimize the opportunities for exposure both to infectious agents and to foreign bodies, such as bones or wrappers, which when ingested may cause gastrointestinal upset or even obstruction.

Summary

Dog walking is an enjoyable and health promoting activity for both people and dogs provided that the safety and welfare of the dog is also addressed. For dogs, in addition to the mental and physical stimulation walking provides, the exercise attained can be a hugely beneficial way to keep dogs fit and/or as part of a weight loss program supervised by a veterinarian.

Overweight and obesity are prevalent in both humans and dogs, and reports suggest that these conditions are becoming more common. Numerous risk factors for overweight or obesity have been described for dogs; many of these risk factors are similar in both humans and dogs. Common risk factors include a calorie-dense diet, over-use of treats, and reduced exercise. Overweight or obesity are also associated with serious medical diseases, including cardiovascular and musculoskeletal disease. Most significantly, dogs that are overweight or obese have a significantly reduced lifespan compared to dogs that maintain a healthy body condition over the course of their life. Effective weight reduction and maintenance of an optimum body condition depends on many factors, but careful attention to diet, exercise, and regular monitoring as part of a coordinated weight management program offers the best of a healthy life for both pet and owner.

Notes

1. Banfield, The Pet Hospital, is a multi-hospital general veterinary practice that began in 1993 in Portland, Oregon with over 750 hospitals in 43 states of the United States. Most locations are housed inside PetSmart stores and all hospitals use the same proprietary electronic health and management system, PetWare,™ to capture client information, medical data, and financial transactions. PetWare™ data are transferred daily to a central server at the corporate headquarters in Portland. On average, more than 115,000 pets are seen per week; the majority are dogs and cats with a small percentage of other species (ferrets, rabbits, reptiles, pocket pets, and birds). Coded medical data captured in PetWare™ includes exam findings, laboratory results, diagnoses, treatments, and client/pet demographics.

References

Avenell, A., Broom, J., Brown, T. J., Poobalan, A., Aucott, L., Stearns, S. C., et al. (2004). Systematic review of the long-term effects and economic consequences of treatments for obesity and implications for health improvement. *Health Technology Assessment, 8*(21), iii-iv, 1-182.

Bauman, A. E., Russell, S. J., Furber, S. E., & Dobson, A. J. (2001). The epidemiology of dog walking: An unmet need for human and canine health. *Medical Journal of Australia, 175*(11-12), 632-634.

Bland, I. M., Guthrie-Jones, A., Taylor, R. D., Hill, J. (2009). Dog obesity: Owner attitudes and behaviour. *Preventative Veterinary Medicine, 92*(4), 333-340.

Bradshaw, J. W. S., & Lea, A. M. (1992). Dyadic interactions between domestic dogs. *Anthrozoos, 5,* 245-253.

Chauvet, A., Laclai, J., Elliott, D. A., & German, A. J. (2010). Incorporation of exercise, using an underwater treadmill, and active client education into a weight management program for obese dogs. *Canadian Veterinary Journal,* in press.

Courcier E .A., Thomson R. M., Mellor D. J., Yam P. S. (2010). An epidemiological study of environmental factors associated with canine obesity. *Journal of Small Animal Practice.* Apr 6 (e-publication ahead of print).

Cutt, H., Giles-Corti, B., Knuiman, M., Timperio, A., & Bull, F. (2008). Understanding dog owners' increased levels of physical activity: Results from RESIDE. *American Journal of Public Health, 98*(1), 66-69.

Defra. (2009). *Code of practice for the welfare of dog*s. London: Defra.

Diez, M., Nguyen, P., Jeusette, I., Devois, C., Istasse, L., & Biourge, V. (2002). Weight loss in obese dogs: Evaluation of a high-protein, low-carbohydrate diet. *Journal of Nutrition, 132*(6 Suppl 2), 1685S-1687S.

Flegal, K. M., Carroll, M. D., Ogden, C. L., & Johnson, C. L. (2002). Prevalence and trends in obesity among US adults, 1999-2000. *Journal of the American Medical Association, 288*(14), 1723-1727.

German, A. J. (2006). The growing problem of obesity in dogs and cats. *Journal of Nutrition, 136*(7 Suppl), 1940S-1946S.

German, A. J., Holden, S. L., Bissot, T., Hackett, R. M., & Biourge, V. (2007). Dietary energy restriction and successful weight loss in obese client-owned dogs. *Journal of Veterinary Internal Medicine, 21*(6), 1174-1180.

German A. J., Morgan L. E. (2008). How often do veterinarians assess the bodyweight and body condition of dogs? *Veterinary Record, Oct 25, 163*(17), 503-505.

German, A. J., Holden, S. L., Bissot, T., Morris, P. J., & Biourge, V. (2007). A high protein high fibre diet improves weight loss in obese dogs. *Veterinary Journal, 183*(3), 294-297.

Gossellin, J., McKelvie, J., Sherington, J., Wren, J. A., Eagleson, J. S., Rowan, T. G., et al. (2007). An evaluation of dirlotapide to reduce body weight of client-owned dogs in two placebo-controlled clinical studies in Europe. *Journal of Veterinary Pharmacological Therapy, 30 Supplement 1*, 73-80.

Gossellin, J., Peachey, S., Sherington, J., Rowan, T. G., & Sunderland, S. J. (2007). Evaluation of dirlotapide for sustained weight loss in overweight Labrador retrievers. *Journal of Veterinary Pharmacolological Therapy, 30 Supplement 1*, 55-65.

Greene, C. E. (2006). Environmental factors in infectious disease. In C. E. Greene (Ed.), *Infectious diseases of the dog and cat* (pp. 991-1013). St Louis: Saunders Elsevier.

Hill, R. C. (2009). Conference on "multidisciplinary approaches to nutritional problems." Symposium on "nutrition and health." Nutritional therapies to improve health: Lessons from companion animals. *Proceedings of the Nutrition Society, 68*(1), 98-102.

Houston, D. K., Nicklas, B. J., & Zizza, C. A. (2009). Weighty concerns: The growing prevalence of obesity among older adults. *Journal of the American Dietetic Association, 109*(11), 1886-1895.

Jewell, D. E., & Toll, P. W. (1996). Effects of fibre on food intake in dogs. *Veterinary Clinical Nutrition*(3), 115-118.

Kealy, R. D., Lawler, D. F., Ballam, J. M., Lust, G., Biery, D. N., Smith, G. K., & Mantz, S. L. (2000). Evaluation of the effect of limited food consumption on radiographic evidence of osteoarthritis in dogs. *Journal of the American Veterinary Medical Association, 217*(11), 1678-1680.

Kienzle, E., Bergler, R., & Mandernach, A. (1998). A comparison of the feeding behavior and the human-animal relationship in owners of normal and obese dogs. *Journal of Nutrition, 128*(12 Suppl), 2779S-2782S.

Kolonin, M. G., Saha, P. K., Chan, L., Pasqualini, R., & Arap, W. (2004). Reversal of obesity by targeted ablation of adipose tissue. *Natural Medicine, 10*(6), 625-632.

Kronfeld, D. S., Donoghue, S., & Glickman, L. T. (1991). Body condition and energy intakes of dogs in a referral teaching hospital. *Journal of Nutrition, 121*(11 Suppl), S157-158.

Laflamme, D. P. (1997). Development and validation of a body condition score system for dogs. *Canine Practice, 22*, 10-15.

Laflamme, D. P. (2006). Understanding and managing obesity in dogs and cats. *Veterinary Clinics of North America Small Animal Practice, 36*(6), 1283-1295, vii.

Linder, D. E., & Freeman, L. M. (2010). Evaluation of calorie density and feeding directions for commercially available diets designed for weight loss in dogs and cats. *Journal of the American Veterinary Medical Association, 236*(1), 74-77.

Lund, E. (2006). Prevalence and risk factors for obesity in adult dogs from private US veterinary practices. *International Journal of Applied Research in Veterinary Medicine, 4*(2), 177-186.

Lund, E. M. (2007). Overweight pets: What's the big deal. *Banfield Journal, 3*(1), 16-20. Retrieved June 15, 2010, from http://www.banfield.net/journal-archive/2007/jan-feb-2007/03-overweight-pets-whats-the-big-deal.pdf

Lund, E. M., Armstrong, P. J., Kirk, C. A., Kolar, L. M., & Klausner, J. S. (1999). Health status and population characteristics of dogs and cats examined at private veterinary practices in the United States. *Journal of the American Veterinary Medical Association, 214*(9), 1336-1341.

Mazzafero, E. (2010). Heatstroke. In S. Ettinger & E. C. Feldman (Eds.), *Textbook of internal medicine* (pp. 509-512). Philadelphia: W. B. Saunders.

McGreevy, P. D., Thomson, P. C., Pride, C., Fawcett, A., Grassi, T., & Jones, B. (2005). Prevalence of obesity in dogs examined by Australian veterinary practices and the risk factors involved. *Veterinary Record, 156*(22), 695-702.

Ogden, C. L., Carroll, M. D., Curtin, L. R., McDowell, M. A., Tabak, C. J., & Flegal, K. M. (2006). Prevalence of overweight and obesity in the United States, 1999-2004. *Journal of the American Medical Association, 295*(13), 1549-1555.

Center for Disease Control (2009). The health effects of overweight and obesity. Retrieved from http://www.cdc.gov/healthyweight/effects/index.html

Rohlf, V., Toukhsati, S, Coleman, G and Bennett, P. (2010) Dog obesity: Can dog caregivers' (owners') feeding and exercise intentions and behaviors be predicted from attitudes? *Journal of Applied Animal Welfare Science, 13*, 213-236.

Roudebush, P., Schoenherr, W. D., & Delaney, S. J. (2008). An evidence-based review of the use of therapeutic foods, owner education, exercise, and drugs for the management of obese and overweight pets. *Journal of the American Veterinary Medical Association, 233*(5), 717-725.

Weber, M., Bissot, T., Servet, E., Sergheraert, R., Biourge, V., & German, A. J. (2007). A high-protein, high-fiber diet designed for weight loss improves satiety in dogs. *Journal Veterinary Internal Medicine, 21*(6), 1203-1208.

Westgarth, C., Christley, R. M., Pinchbeck, G. L., Gaskell, R. M., Dawson, S., & Bradshaw, J. W. (2010). Dog behaviour on walks and the effect of use of the leash. *Applied Animal Behaviour Science, 125*(1), 38-46.

Westgarth, C., Porter, C. J., Nicolson, L., Birtles, R. J., Williams, N. J., Hart, C. A., et al. (2009). Risk factors for the carriage of Campylobacter upsaliensis by dogs in a community in Cheshire. *Veterinary Record, 165*(18), 526-530.

Wren, J. A., Ramudo, A. A., Campbell, S. L., King, V. L., Eagleson, J. S., Gossellin, J., et al. (2007). Efficacy and safety of dirlotapide in the management of obese dogs evaluated in two placebo-controlled, masked clinical studies in North America. *Journal Veterinary Pharmacological Therapy, 30 Supplement 1*, 81-89.

Yaissle, J. E., Holloway, C., Buffington, C. A. (2004). Evaluation of owner education as a component of obesity treatment programs for dogs. *Journal of the American Veterinary Medical Association, Jun 15, 224*(12),1932-1935.

Chapter 9

Owners and pets exercising together: The metabolic benefits of "walking the dog"

Mark B. Stephens, Cindy C. Wilson, Jeffrey L. Goodie, F. Ellen Netting, Cara Olsen, Christopher G. Byers, and Mary E. Yonemura

Background and significance

The health impact of overweight and obesity

Two out of every three American adults are either overweight or obese (Flegal, 2010). Studies indicate the trend of increasing obesity in United States adults began sometime after the Civil War and has accelerated in recent decades before stabilizing in the past several years (Flegal, 2010; Costa, 1997). In the U.S., the trend of rising obesity is not limited to adults. The number of obese children has risen more than threefold in the past several decades as well (Ogden, 2008). In fact, it is predicted that if current trends of overweight continue, for the first time in modern history the current generation of American children will have a shorter life expectancy than their parents (Olshansky, 2005). This decline in life expectancy is anticipated due to well-known comorbidities associated with overweight and obesity including cardiovascular disease, diabetes, dyslipidemia, and hypertension, which increase mortality (Mokdad, 2004). Numerous public health efforts to combat the rise in overweight and obesity have been proposed in the past several decades (*Healthy People 2020*, Surgeon General). At an estimated cost of $147 billion per year (Finkelstein, 2009), morbidity associated with overweight and obesity remains one of the top public health challenges facing the worldwide medical community for the foreseeable future.

Obesity is not confined to human populations

Paralleling the rise in human obesity is a rise in canine obesity (Lund, 2006). Dogs are overweight when they exceed 15% of ideal weight, and obese when their bodyweight exceeds 30% of ideal (Gosselin, 2007). Studies estimate the prevalence of overweight/obesity in the dog population to range between 22% and 40% (McGreevy, 2005; Colliard, 2006). Other cross-sectional data suggest one in three dogs seen by U.S. veterinarians is overweight (German, 2006). As in humans, obesity in dogs has been linked with a variety of diseases including diabetes, lipid disorders, and orthopedic maladies (German, 2006). Not surprisingly, the same risk factors of physical inactivity and poor nutrition (Bland, 2009) that have led to human obesity have also led to the growing prevalence of obesity in dogs (Laflamme, 2006).

In this chapter, a brief overview of the factors involved in human and canine overweight and obesity will be provided in the context of examining the potential for human-animal interaction to serve as an intervention for addressing this problem in human and canine populations. Studies concerning physical activity in the human-animal relationship are reviewed along with preliminary results from the Owners and Pets Exercising Together (OPET) project. Implications for further research are provided.

Metabolic factors associated with adipose and disease: All fat is not equal

Humans have two primary types of adipose tissue: brown fat and white fat. Brown fat plays a role in thermogenesis and is believed to be less important in the development of metabolic disease. White fat is stored either as subcutaneous or as visceral fat. Long felt to be an inert bystander in overweight patients, current research reveals white fat to be a dynamic metabolic organ centrally involved in the pathogenesis of morbidities associated with overweight and obesity (Weiss, 2005). Visceral white fat is an active participant in the pathogenesis of disease associated with overweight and obesity in humans (Mathieu, 2010) and in canines (Axelsson, 2005). In humans, the distribution of visceral fat impacts disease risk. Specifically, measures of central obesity more accurately correlate with metabolic risk than do measures of peripheral adiposity such as skin folds (Bosy-Westphal, 2006). Individuals with an "apple" shape have more cardiovascular events and worse outcomes than do those with a "pear" physique (Reis, 2009).

Visceral fat is an active participant in tissue inflammation, metabolic syndrome, and the continuum of cardiovascular risk in humans and in canines (Eisele, 2005). Visceral adipose tissue secretes a series of peptides known as adipocytokines. These peptides, in turn, mediate the development of metabolic syndrome by modulating levels of local tissue inflammation. One adipocyto-kine in particular, adiponectin, appears to play a protective role in the patho-genesis of the metabolic syndrome. Specifically, adiponectin exerts an anti-inflammatory effect by inhibiting the secretion of tumor necrosis factor (TNF), C-reactive protein (CRP), and other inflammatory mediators. Sufficient levels of adiponectin guard against insulin resistance and serve a vasculoprotective role (Szmitko, 2007). Adiponectin levels, however, correlate inversely with visceral fat levels. As visceral fat levels increase and levels of adiponectin fall, secretion of pro-inflammatory mediators such as TNF and CRP increases, leading to local tissue inflammation (Valle, 2005; Patel, 2006). Local tissue inflammation then contributes to the development of insulin resistance, abnor-malities in serum lipids, and hypertension. This phenomenon clinically reveals itself as the metabolic syndrome. Although some of the specific inflammatory markers associated with inflammation, cardiovascular disease, and the meta-bolic syndrome are either expensive or difficult to measure, other parameters lend themselves well to measurement for screening purposes.

Current guidelines call for routine screening of a variety of metabolic factors to assess the impact that visceral fat may be having on an individual's risk of disease and determine the best course of treatment. The U.S. Preventive Services Task Force recommends expanded screening for obesity (USPSTF, 2010), diabetes (USPSTF, 2010), and lipid disorders (USPSTF, 2010) within the general population.

Body mass index and body condition score

The body mass index (BMI) is the most commonly used tool for classifying humans as overweight or obese (BMI=weight [kg]/height [m]^2). Adults are defined as underweight (BMI<18.5), normal (BMI=18.5-24.9), overweight (BMI=25-29.9), obese (BMI=30-39.9), or extreme obesity (BMI≥40). In adult humans, an increased BMI is associated with increased risk for cardiovas-cular disease, certain cancers, diabetes, and overall mortality (Guh, 2009; Shizamu, 2009).

For canines, one means of assessing weight status is the body condition score (BCS). The BCS is a simple, noninvasive tool for assessing canine obesity during a complete physical examination (Dorsten, 2004), and provides a sub-jective yet quantitative way to estimate the amount of excess adipose present. Using the validated, 9-point Laflamme system, each point represents approximately 10% to 15% of body weight. Overweight is defined as 6 or 7 on 9-point scale, whereas obesity is defined as 8 or more (Laflamme, 1997). Longitudinal recording of both body weight and BCS allows veterinary health professionals to more easily provide weight and nutritional counseling to owners about their dog through serial monitoring of trends in canine obesity (German, 2009).

Glucose

Overweight and obesity are independent risk factors for the development of type 2 diabetes. Obesity contributes to insulin resistance (Kahn, 2000) that in turn increases circulating blood glucose levels leading to diabetes. Diabetes is associated with increased cardiovascular disease (Kannel, 1979) and premature mortality (Morgan, 2000). There is less convincing data that obesity is an independent risk factor for canine diabetes (Rand, 2004).

Cholesterol and serum lipoproteins

Cholesterol is important for development and functioning of cell membranes. It has long been known that elevations in the levels of total cholesterol are associated with heart disease in humans (Wilson, 1998). Cholesterol is transported through the bloodstream by lipoprotein particles that further contribute to the development of heart disease. Although many new lipoproteins are constantly being identified, traditional serum lipid measurements include:

1. *Low Density Lipoproteins (LDL).* Referred to as "bad cholesterol" in lay terms, LDL is atherogenic. LDL transports cholesterol to cells (including vascular endothelium), contributing to the development of plaques and atherosclerosis (Grundy, 1995).

2. *High Density Lipoproteins (HDL).* In contrast to LDL, HDL ("good cholesterol") transports cholesterol away from cells to the liver for metabolism and excretion. High serum levels of HDL appear to be cardioprotective and reduce the risk of heart disease (Barter, 2005). Individuals who are obese are known to have high-risk lipid profiles including both cholesterol and lipoprotein fractions, perhaps mediated through elevated levels of adipocytokines and free fatty acids associated with increasing levels of visceral fat (Gade, 2010).

3. *Triglycerides.* Most of the fats that humans digest are triglycerides. Triglycerides have recently been identified as an independent risk factor for heart disease, particularly when associated with low levels of HDL (McBride, 2008). In experimental populations, plasma levels of triglycerides and LDL increase with body weight in obese canines as well (Jeusette, 2006).

Physical activity and health

Of major concern in the current obesity epidemic are increasing sedentary behaviors among the general public. In addition to reducing all cause mortality, regular physical activity (PA) helps prevent chronic diseases such as coronary artery disease and diabetes mellitus (Warburton, 2006). Regular PA reduces the incidence of disabling diseases such as osteoporosis and arthritis while reducing risk factors for chronic disease such as hypertension and high cholesterol (Fletcher, 1996).

Despite the recognized benefits of physical activity, fewer than half of adults engage in recommended levels of exercise (Sapkota, 2005). In data tracked since 1997, the National Health Interview Study (NHIS) estimates only 30% of adults engage in sufficient leisure time physical activity and that nearly 25% of adults do not participate in any leisure time activity at all (CDC, 2010). Similarly, one community-based study suggests more than half of all dog owners do not walk their dogs at all (Bauman, 2001). Sedentary behaviors contribute adversely to the health burden of owners and their companion animals.

To help combat growing trends in canine obesity, the Humane Society of the United States recommends twice daily walking to improve canine health and fitness (HSA, 2010). The federal government has released physical activity guidelines recommending Americans accumulate a minimum of 150 minutes of moderate-intensity physical activity per week (DHHS, 2008). Given the large proportion of households that own a dog, increasing simple dog walking may have significant health benefits for owners as well as their canine companions (Ham, 2006).

Pet ownership and health

The health benefits of pet ownership (PO) appear to have a positive impact on leading health indicators such as diabetes mellitus, physical activity, nutrition, and weight status targeted in *Healthy People 2020*. Multiple areas such as diabetes mellitus, heart disease, physical activity, fitness, nutrition, and overweight are positively influenced by PO and argue strongly for collaboration between veterinary and human medicine in a One Health model to combat multiple diseases impacting humans and animals (King, 2008).

There are roughly 75 million pet dogs in the U.S. (AVMA, 2007), equating to nearly 40% of all households. Eighty five percent of these dog owners will visit a veterinarian with their dog at least once a year. Most dog owners consider their animal to be part of the family. As such, dog ownership has been shown to confer significant health benefits on their owners (Jennings, 1997). Dog owners report fewer minor health issues and engage in more recreational walks than non-owners (Yabroff, 2008). Owning a companion dog increases the spontaneous physical activity level in most adults (Coleman, 2008; Cutt, 2008). As one example, the National Household Travel Survey (NHTS), a cross-sectional survey of personal transportation by the civilian, non-institutionalized population in the U.S., examined the number of walking trips by dog owners for the purpose of pet care (Ham, 2006). Among dog walkers, 80% of owners walked their animal a minimum of 10 minutes each day. Nearly two-thirds took their animal for two or more walks per day. Nearly half of the adults in the sample who walked their dog two or three times a day easily accumulated 30 minutes or more of walking in a day. This level of physical activity contributes to the overall fitness for both the dogs and their owners. In general, dog owners are more physically active than non-owners (Thorpe, 2006).

Dog walking may also add to human health benefits by creating a form of social support and perceived obligation contributing to increased physical activity (Bryant, 1985; Wood, 2005). A large body of research supports the positive health effects of human companionship (Beck, 1996). The health benefits of having a companion animal are well described and transcend race and culture (Ham, 2006; Risley-Curtiss, 2006). Pets serve as a source of social support (Serpell, 1991), bolster their companion's sense of competence and self-worth (Wells, 2007), and provide the opportunity for shared pleasure in spontaneous recreation and relaxation (McNicholas, 2005). Data from the RESIDE Study in Australia suggest individuals are more likely to regularly adhere to a walking program after obtaining a dog (Cutt, 2008). The dog is a companion with whom the owner exercises. Walking with a dog is convenient, requires no special equipment, and may be done at any time within one's own locale.

Current gaps in the literature

Developing effective methods for increasing the physical activity of the population is an important step toward continuing to reverse overweight and obesity trends and improves the metabolic factors that impact the course of disease. A review of multiple interventions for increasing physical activity (e.g., community-wide campaigns, mass media campaigns, family-based social support) suggests individually-adapted health behavior change programs are among the most successful at increasing physical activity (Kahn, 2002). It is unfortunate that only 34% of patients seen for a medical checkup report being counseled about their physical activity (Wee, 1999). There is mixed evidence about whether counseling to increase physical activity by medical providers results in sustained behavior changes (Eden, 2002). Leveraging the unique relationship between owners and their dogs to facilitate increased physical activity may enhance the likelihood owners engage in more activity and improve the health of both themselves and their dog. Community-based veterinarians, therefore, play an intriguing role in potentially addressing the issue of both human and canine obesity.

The OPET study: Metabolic benefits of "walking the dog"

Study design

The Owners and Pets Exercising Together (OPET) study examines biopsychosocial relations between owners and their dogs and whether physical activity counseling for the dog provided by a specialty-care veterinarian impacts physical activity levels and the metabolic status of owners and their dogs. Dog owners attending a clinical appointment for their dog are asked to participate in the study. Interested participants are asked to complete a self-report survey of demographic information and have their body mass index assessed. Their dog's somatotype is then assessed using the 9-point Laflamme BCS (Laflamme 1997). If the BCS of the dog is 6 or greater, indicating the dog is overweight or obese, the pet owner is asked to participate in the second phase of the study. In phase 2, additional self-report measures are completed, and blood samples from both the owner and their dog are analyzed for specific metabolic components.

Using a randomized-controlled trial design, the OPET study is designed to examine the impact of veterinarian-directed physical activity counseling on human and canine measures of chronic disease. Veterinarians provide specific counseling designed to increase opportunities for dogs and (by secondary intention) their owners. Eligible participants are randomly assigned to one of two interventions, a "standard care group" or a "physical activity group." Both groups have blood drawn for glucose and lipid measurements. A baseline assessment of physical activity using a pedometer is performed in both groups as well. Participants randomized to the "standard care group" meet with the veterinarian as part of their scheduled appointment and review general preventive health care for their dog. This standard script includes generic canine wellness information, oral health, disease prevention, nutrition guidelines, and generic recommendations regarding physical activity. No specific activity goals are discussed in the standard care group. Participants randomized to the "physical activity group" receive specific exercise counseling from a veterinarian to specifically increase their dog's physical activity levels. This is in addition to the general wellness information received by the standard care participants.

Owners in the activity group are actively encouraged to ensure that their dog accumulates a minimum 30 minutes of physical activity a day. Owners are then given a pedometer to wear and are asked to record the times they are engaged in physical activity with their dog on a daily basis. After three months, owners and dogs in both groups have repeat samples taken for glucose and lipid measurements and return to the clinic to have the dog's BCS assessed, the owner's BMI measured, and owners complete all self-report measures associated with the study.

Preliminary findings from the OPET study

Preliminary data from the prospective OPET study were presented at the 18th annual conference of the International Society for Anthrozoology in Kansas City, Missouri. Forty pets owners had enrolled in the study, and 28 had completed the study at that time. The mean age of the dogs was 7.0 years (SD=3.9 years). Mean BCS of the 28 dogs in Phase I was 5.98 +/- 1.17. Among the 12 dogs that had complete data for phase 1 and phase 2, their mean BCS was 6.58 +/- 0.67 at phase 1, and their mean BCS at the end of phase 2 was 6.17 +/- 0.94. On average, body condition score decreased by 0.26 (a 4% change) and weight decreased by 1.2 lbs (a 2.4% change). Of the 28 pet owners who had enrolled in phase 2, 16% (n=?) dropped out for reasons that included declining health on the part of the dog, failure to follow study protocol, and other logistical challenges. For humans, despite a slight increase in BMI, participating dog owners demonstrate modest average decreases (2% to 5%) in glucose, cholesterol, triglycerides, and LDL from baseline. Because data collection is ongoing, we are as yet blinded to the intervention status of individual participants (Table 9.1).

Implications and future directions

Although data from the human literature suggest primary care physicians have an obligation to counsel sedentary and overweight patients to increase their level of physical activity (Chakravarthy, 2002), similar findings are not available in the veterinary literature. The preliminary findings from the OPET study suggest counseling conducted by a veterinarian to increase physical activity levels in their canine patients may have an important metabolic "spillover" effect on owners as well. Although the early findings in the OPET study are modest, final enrollment data analysis is ongoing to a target accrual of 75 human-canine dyads. Our study supports a growing body of literature extolling the health benefits of walking the dog. The OPET study focuses specifically on glucose and lipoprotein homeostasis. A larger trial examining the impact of dog walking on other metabolic markers of inflammation (adiponectin, C-reactive protein, and other inflammatory cytokines) and visceral fat homeostasis using the OPET study design is in the initial stages as well. The potential of the family veterinarian as a member of the health care team has merit for a community-based program promoting physical activity and weight loss.

Table 9.1. Demographic and metabolic data from 24 human participants in the OPET study (Stephens, 2010).

Variable	Study Period	Mean	Std Dev	Minimum	Maximum
Glucose	baseline	98.7	24.9	54	161
	follow-up	96.9	21.2	75	159
Cholesterol	baseline	185.5	30.6	144	259
	follow-up	180.7	23.4	131	234
Triglycerides	baseline	125.7	68.6	44	275
	follow-up	119.9	78.6	49	366
HDL	baseline	61.4	17.8	35	93
	follow-up	61.5	19.2	37	96
LDL	baseline	99.0	31.8	36	181
	follow-up	95.2	25.8	51	139
BMI	baseline	28.7			
	follow-up	28.9			
Age		43.6	15.5	18	73
Female gender		90%			

Note: HDL=high density lipoprotein; LDL=low density lipoprotein; BMI=body mass index

Disclaimer

Project funded by a grant from the Waltham® Centre for Pet Nutrition. The opinions contained herein are those of the authors. They do not represent official policy of the Department of the Navy, the Public Health Service, the Uniformed Services University, or the Department of Defense.

References

American Veterinary Medical Association. (2007). US pet ownership & demographics sourcebook.

Axelsson, J., Heimburger, O., Lindholm, B., & Stenvinkel, P. (2005). Adipose tissue and its relation to inflammation: The role of adipokines. *Journal of Renal Nutrition, 15*, 131-136

Barter, P. J. (2005). Cardioprotective effects of high-density lipoproteins: The evidence strengthens. *Arterioscerosis, Thrombosis, and Vascular Biology, 25*, 1305.

Bauman, A. E., Russell, S. J., Furber, S. E., & Dobson, A. J. (2001). The epidemiology of dog walking: An unmet need for human and canine health. *Medical Journal of Australia, 175*(11-12), 632-634

Beck, A. M., & Meyers, N. M. (1996). Health enhancement and companion animal ownership. *Annul Reviews Public Health, 17*, 247-257.

Bland, I. M., Guthrie-Jones, A., Taylor, R. D, & Hill, J. (2009). Dog obesity: Owner attitudes and behaviour. *Preventive Veterinary Medicine, 92*, 333-340.

Bosy-Westphal, A., Geisler, C., Onur, S., Korth, O., Selberg, O., Schrezenmeir, S., & Muller, M. J. (2006). Value of body fat mass vs. anthropometric obesity indices in the assessment of metabolic risk factors. *International Journal of Obesity (London), 30*(3), 475-483.

Bryant, B. K. (1985). The neighborhood walk: Sources of support in middle childhood. *Monographs of the Society for Research in Child Development, 50*, No. 3.

Caring for your dog: the top ten essentials. Washington, DC: The Humane Society of the United States. Retrieved April 17, 2010, from http://www.humanesociety.org/animals/dogs/tips/dog_care_essentials.html

Centers for Disease Control and Prevention. National Health Interview Study. Retrieved April 27, 2010, from http://www.cdc.gov/nchs/data/nhis/earlyrelease/201003_07.pdf

Chakravarthy, M.V., Joyner, M. J., & Booth, F.W. (2002). An obligation for primary care physicians to prescribe physical activity to sedentary patients to reduce the risk of chronic health conditions. *Mayo Clinic Proceedings, 77*(2), 165-173.

Coleman, K. J., Rosenberg, D. E., Conway, T. L., Sallis, J. F. Saelens, B. E., Frank, L. D., & Cain, K. (2008). Physical activity, weight status, and neighborhood characteristics of dog walkers. *Preventive Veterinary Medicine, 47*(3), 309-312.

Colliard, L., Ancel, J., Benet, J. J., Paragon, B. M., & Blanchard, G. (2006). Risk factors for obesity in dogs in France. *The Journal of Nutrition, 136*, 1951S-1954S.

Costa, D. L., & Steckel, R. H. (1997). Long-term trends in health, welfare, and economic growth in the United States. In R. H. Steckel & R. Floud (Eds.), *Health and welfare during industrialization* (pp. 47-49). Chicago, IL: The University of Chicago Press.

Cutt, H. E., Knuiman, M. W., & Giles-Corti, B. (2008). Does getting a dog increase recreational walking? *International Journal of Behavioral Nutrition and Physical Activity*, 5, 17-24.

Cutt, H. E., Giles-Corti, B., Wood, L. J., Knuiman, M. W., & Burke, V. (2008). Barriers and motivators for owners walking their dog: Results from qualitative research. *Health Promotion Journal of Australia*, 19(2), 118-124.

Dorsten, C. M., & Cooper, D. M. (2004). Use of body condition scoring to manage body weight in dogs. *Contemporary Topics in Laboratory Animal Science*, 43, 34-37.

Eden, K. B., Orleans, C. T., Mulrow, C. D., Pender, N. J., & Teutsch, S. M. (2002). Does counseling by clinicians improve physical activity? A summary of the evidence for the U.S. Preventive Services Task Force. *Annals of Internal Medicine*, 137(3), 208-215.

Eisele, I., Wood, I. S., German, A. J., Hunter, L., & Trayhum, P. (2005). Adipokine gene expression in dog adipose tissues and dog white adipocytes differentiated in primary culture. *Hormone and Metabolic Research*, 37, 474-481.

Finkelstein, E. A., Trogdon, J., C., Cohen, J. W., & Dietz, W. (2009). Annual medical spending attributable to obesity: Payer and service-specific estimates. *Health Affairs (Millwood)*, 28(5), w822-w831.

Flegal, K. M., Carroll, M. D., Ogden, C. L., & Curtin, L. R. (2010). Prevalence and trends in obesity among US adults, 1999-2008. *Journal of the American Medical Association*, 303(3), 235-241.

Fletcher, G. F., Balady, G., Blair, S. N., Blumentha, J., Caspersen, C., Chaitman, B., Epstein, S., Sivarajan Froelicher, E. S,. Froelicher, V. F, Pina, I. L., & Pollock, M. L. (1996). Statement on exercise: Benefits and recommendations for physical activity programs for all Americans. *Circulation*, 94, 857-862.

Gade, W., Schmit, J., Collins, M., & Gade, J. (2010). Beyond obesity: The diagnosis and pathophysiology of metabolic syndrome. *Clinical Laboratory Science*, 23(1), 51-61.

German, A. J., Holden, S. L., Bissot, T., Morris, P.J., & Biourge, V. (2009). Use of starting condition score to estimate changes in body weight and composition during weight loss in obese dogs. *Research in Veterinary Science*, 87, 49-254.

German, A. J. (2006). The growing problem of obesity in dogs and cats. *The Journal of Nutrition*, 136(7 Suppl), 1940S-1946S.

Gossellin, J., & Wren, J. A. (2007). Sunderland SJ: Canine obesity: An overview. *Journal of Veterinary Pharmacology and Therapeutics, 30* Suppl 1-10.

Grundy, S. M. (1995). Role of low-density lipoproteins in atherogenesis and development of coronary heart disease. *Clinical Chemistry, 41*, 139-146.

Guh, D. P., Zhang, W., Bansback, N., Amarisi, Z., Birmingham, C. L., & Anis, A. H. (2009). The incidence of co-morbidities related to obesity and overweight: A systematic review and meta-analysis. *BMC Public Health, 25*(9), 88-96.

Ham, S. A., Epping, J. (2006) Dog walking and physical activity in the United States. *Preventing Chronic Disease, 3*(2), A46.

Healthy People 2020. Retrieved May 27, 2010, from http://www.healthypeople. gov/hp2020/Objectives/TopicAreas.aspx

Jennings, L. B. (1997). Potential benefits of pet ownership in health promotion. *Journal of Holistic Nursing, 15*(4), 358-372.

Jeusette, I. C., Lhoest, E.T., Istasse, L.P., & Diez, M. O. (2005). Influence of obesity on plasma lipid and lipoprotein concentrations in dogs. *American Journal of Veterinary Research, 66*, 81-86.

Kahn, B. B., & Flier, J. S. (2000). Obesity and insulin resistance. *The Journal of Clinical Investigation, 106*(4), 473-481.

Kahn, E. B., Ramsey, L. T., Brownson, R. C., Heath, G. W., Howze, E. H., Powell, K. E., Stone, E. J., Rajab, M. W., Corso, P., & the Task Force on Community Preventive Services. (2002). The effectiveness of interventions to increase physical activity: A systematic review. *American Journal of Preventive Medicine, 22*(4S), 73-107.

Kannel, W. B., & McGee, D. L. (1979). Diabetes and cardiovascular disease. *Journal of the American Medical Association, 241*(19), 2035-2038.

King, L. J., Anderson, L. R., & Blackmore, C.G. (2008). Executive summary of the AVMA One Health initiative task force. *Journal of the American Veterinary Medical Association, 233*(2), 259-261

Laflamme, D. P. (1997). Development and validation of a body condition score system for dogs. *Canine Practice, 22*(July-August), 10–5.12.

Laflamme, D. P. (2006). Understanding and managing obesity in dogs and cats. *Veterinary Clinics of North America: Small Animal Practice, 36*, 1283-1295.

Lund, E. M., Armstrong, P. J., Kirk, C. A., & Klausner, J. S. (2006). Prevalence and risk factors for obesity in adult dogs from private US veterinary practices. *International Journal of Applied Research in Veterinary Medicine, 4*(2), 177-186.

Mathieu, P., Lemieux, I., & Després, J. P. (2010). Obesity, inflammation and cardiovascular risk. *Clinical Pharmacology Therapeutics, 87*(4), 407-416.

McBride, P. (2008). Triglycerides and risk for coronary artery disease. *Current Atherosclerosis Reports, 10*(5), 386-390.

McGreevy, P. D., Thomson, P. C., Pride, C., Fawcett, A., Grassi, T., & Jones, B. (2005). Prevalence of obesity in dogs examined by Australian veterinary practices and the risk factors involved. *Veterinary Record, 156*(22), 695-702.

McNicholas, J., Gilbey, A., Rennie, A., Ahmedzai, S., Dono, J., & Ormerod, E. (2005). Pet ownership and human health: A brief review of evidence and issues. *British Medical Journal, 331*, 1252-1254.

Mokdad, A. H., Marks, J. S., Stroup, D. F., & Gerberding, J. L. (2004). Actual causes of death in the United States. *The Journal of the American Medical Association, 291*, 1238-1245.

Morgan, C., L., Currie, C. J., & Peters, J. R. (2000). Relationship between diabetes and mortality: A population study using record linkage. *Diabetes Care, 23*(8), 1103-1107.

Ogden, C. L., Carroll, M. D., & Flegal, K .M. (2008). High body mass index for age among US children and adolescents, 2003–2006. *The Journal of the American Medical Association, 299*(20), 2401-2405.

Olshansky, S. J., Passaro, D. J., & Hershow, R. C. (2005). A potential decline in life expectancy in the United States in the 21st century. *New England Journal of Medicine, 352*, 1138-1145.

Patel, D. A., Srinivasan, S. R., Xu, J. H., Chen, W., & Berenson, G. S. (2006). Adiponectin and its correlates of cardiovascular risk in young adults: The Bogalusa Heart Study. *Metabolism, 55*(11), 1551-1557.

Rand, J. S., Fleeman, L.M., Farrow, H. A., Appleton, D. J., & Lederer, R. (2004). Canine and feline diabetes mellitus: Nature or nurture? *The Journal of Nutrition, 134*, 2072S-2080S.

Reis, J. P., Araneta, M. R., Wingard, D. L., Macera, C. A., Lindsay, S. P., & Marshall, S. J. (2009). Overall obesity and abdominal adiposity as predictors of mortality in US white and black adults. *Annuals of Epidemiology, 19*(2), 134-142.

Risley-Curtiss, C., Holley, L. C., & Wolf, S. (2006). The animal-human bond and ethnic diversity. *Social Work, 51*(3), 257-268.

Sapkota, S., Bowles, H. R., & Ham, S. A. (2005). Adult participation in recommended levels of physical activity-United States, 2001 and 2003. *Morbidity and Mortality Weekly Report, 54*(47), 1208-1212.

Serpell, J. (1991). Beneficial effects of pet ownership on some aspects of human health and behaviour. *Journal of the Royal Society of Medicine, 84*(12), 717-720.

Shizamu, T., Kuriyama, S., Ohmori-Matsuda, K, Kikuchi, N., Nakaya, N., & Tsuji, I. (2009). Increase in body mass index category since age 20 years and all-cause mortality: A prospective cohort study (the Ohasaki Study). *International Journal of Obesity (Lond), 33*(4), 490-496.

Stephens, M. B., Byers, C., Nutting, E., & Wilson, C. Owners and pets exercising together (OPET): The metabolic benefits of walking the dog. NIH Poster Presentation1. International Society of Anthrozoology meeting. Kansas City, MO. October 23, 2009.

Szmitko, P. E., Teoh, H., Stewart, D. J., & Verma, S. (2007). Adiponectin and cardiovascular disease. *American Journal of Physiology - Heart and Circulatory Physiology, 292*, H1655-H1663.

The Surgeon General's call to action to prevent and decrease overweight and obesity. Retrieved April 18, 2010, from www.surgeongeneral.gov/topics/obesity/

Thorpe, R. J., Kreisle, R. A., Glickman, L. T., Simonsick, E. M., Newman, A. B., & Kritchevsky, S. (2006). Physical activity and pet ownership in year 3 of the Health ABC Study. *Journal of Aging and Physical Activity, 14*, 154-168.

U.S. Department of Health and Human Services. Physical Activity Guidelines for Americans, 2008. Retrieved May 27, 2010, from http://www.health.gov/paguidelines/factsheetprof.aspx

U.S. Preventive Services Task Force. Screening for obesity in adults. Retrieved May 27, 2010, from http://www.uspreventiveservicestaskforce.org/uspstf/uspsobes.htm

U.S. Preventive Services Task Force. Screening for diabetes mellitus in adults. Retrieved May 27, 2010, from http://www.uspreventiveservicestaskforce.org/uspstf/uspsdiab.htm

U.S. Preventive Services Task Force. Screening for lipid disorders in adults. Retrieved May 27, 2010, from http://www.uspreventiveservicestaskforce.org/uspstf/uspschol.htm

Valle, M., Martos, R., Gascon, F., et al. (2005). Low-grade systemic inflammation, hypoadiponectinemia and a high concentration of leptin are present in very young obese children, and correlate with metabolic syndrome. *Diabetes Metabolism, 31*, 55-62.

Warburton, D. E. R., Nicol, C. W., & Bredin, S. S. D. (2006). Health benefits of physical activity: The evidence. *Canadian Medical Association Journal, 174*(6), 801-809.

Wee, C. C., McCarthy, E. P., Davis, R. B., & Phillips, R. S. (1999). Physician counseling about exercise. *Journal of the American Veterinary Medical Association, 282*(16), 1583-1588.

Weiss, R., & Caprio, S. (2005). The metabolic consequences of childhood obesity. *Best Practice & Research, 19*(3), 405-419.

Wells, D. L. (2007). Domestic dogs and human health: An overview. *British Journal of Health Psychology, 12*(1), 145-156.

Wilson, P. W. F., D'Agostino, R. B., Levy, D., Belanger, A. M., Silbershatz, H., & Kannel, W. (1998). Prediction of coronary heart disease using risk factor categories. *Circulation, 97*, 1837-1847.

Wood, L., Giles-Corti, B., & Bulsara, M. (2005). The pet connection: Pets as a conduit for social capital? *Social Science & Medicine, 61*(6), 1159-1173.

Yabroff, K. R., & Troiano, R. P. (2008). Walking the dog: Is pet ownership associated with physical activity in California? *Journal of Physical Activity and Health, 5*(2), 216-228.

Chapter 10

Kids and K-9s for healthy choices: A pilot program for canine therapy and healthy behavior modification to increase healthy lifestyle choices in children

Kathy K. Wright and Ashley M. Brown

The prevalence of childhood overweight and obesity in the United States continues to grow to epidemic levels, resulting in a great need for effective health promotion and education programs. It has been shown that promoting and establishing healthy behaviors in children is more effective than efforts to modify unhealthy behaviors in adults (Centers for Disease Control and Prevention, 2010). Health education programs help to address several risk behaviors, such as physical inactivity and unhealthy eating, which are established during childhood and which contribute to the leading causes of death, disability, and social problems in our country (National Center for Chronic Disease Prevention and Health Promotion, 2010).

Between 1976–1980 and 2007–2008, obesity has increased from 6.5% to 19.6% among children aged 6 to 11 and has increased from 5.0% to 18.1% among adolescents aged 12 to 19 here in the United States (CDC, 2004). Complications commonly found in children with obesity include hypertension, type 2 diabetes, depression, and sleep apnea. Obese children and adolescents are more likely to be obese as adults (Whitaker, Wright, Pepe, Seidel, & Dietz, 1997), which makes the implications of childhood obesity on the nation's health and health care costs substantial. Obesity is defined as having a BMI in the 95th or higher percentile; overweight is defined as a BMI in the 85th to 94th percentile (CDC, 2009). BMI is calculated from an individual's height and weight and is an indicator of body fat. Although these measurements are not diagnostic, they are useful in screening for weight categories that may lead to

163

future health conditions. Due to the change in body fat with age and the variances of body fat between males and females, child and adolescent BMIs are best interpreted through BMI-for-age-and-sex growth charts (CDC, 2009).

Physical inactivity has been identified as a contributing factor for childhood obesity. In the last 20 years the number of children in the United States who are physically active has decreased while the number of children who are overweight has doubled (CDC, 2002). American kids spend an average of 5.5 hours per day being physically inactive by engaging in television viewing, playing video games, or using a computer (Roberts & Foehr, 2004). Children and adolescents receive substantial health benefits by achieving recommended activity levels: sixty or more minutes of moderate and vigorous aerobic and age-appropriate muscle and bone strengthening activity every day (United States Department of Health and Human Services, 2008). Physical activity helps build and maintain strong physical health, control weight, lower blood pressure, reduce fat, and improve mental health by building self–esteem (Centers for Disease Control and Prevention, 2002).

Dog walking has recently been studied as a way to increase physical activity. A 2006 study reported that 80.2% of dog owners take at least one 10-minute walk per day with their dog, and 42.3% walk at least 30 minutes with their dog (Ham & Epping, 2006). Kushner (2006) stated that dogs can provide a social support system for dog owners to lose weight because dogs influence important components of social support such as motivation and encouragement. It has been reported that children in dog-owning families have higher levels of physical activity compared with children in non-dog-owning families (Owen et al., 2010). In addition to the physical benefits of dog walking, psychosocial benefits of dog ownership have been identified as well. Dogs help to foster social interactions, influence children's attitudes about themselves, and increase their ability to relate with others (Messent, 1983; Lockwood, 1983). Dog owners have lower risk factors for cardiovascular disease and blood pressure (Anderson et al., 1992) and lower feelings of loneliness and depression (Katcher, 1982; Garrity, Stallions, Marx, & Johnson, 1989). Dogs can fulfill both physical and emotional needs that include physical activity, love, loyalty, and affection (American Academy of Child & Adolescent Psychiatry, 2008). Dog ownership and dog walking, with their array of physical and psychological benefits, could represent a new approach to treating and preventing childhood obesity.

Contributing factors to the childhood overweight and obesity are multifactorial (genetics, environment, lifestyle, and/or cultural), and therefore, prevention strategies should also address these factors through multiple program components. Environmental and behavioral factors leading to obesity have been identified as the "greatest areas for prevention and treatment actions" (CDC, 2009). Behavioral change models offer a framework for understanding health-related behaviors and modifying those behaviors. One such model, the Information-Motivation and Behavioral Skills model (IMB), postulates that health-related information, motivation, and behavioral skills are important determinants of whether or not a health behavior is performed. According to the model, well-informed and well-motivated individuals will apply their behavioral skills to effect a behavior change (Fisher & Fisher, 2002). The model was found to be effective in guiding public health prevention studies, such as understanding HIV risk and prevention (Fisher, Fisher, Bryan, & Miscovich, 2002) and understanding adherence to therapies for self-monitoring blood glucose levels (Bayer Diabetes Care, 2010). In a more broad application, the IMB model could lead to more effective intervention studies and programs designed to modify unhealthy lifestyle behaviors and address the growing trends in childhood obesity. The IMB model served as the structural basis for the content and delivery format used in the "Kids and K-9s for Healthy Choices" program. The program used a combination approach of information-giving, motivation-stimulating, and behavior facilitating methods to increase the understanding and utilization of nutrition and exercise knowledge, to increase physical activity levels, and to facilitate human-dog interactions in school-age children.

Purpose

The purpose of this paper is to describe Kids and K-9s for Healthy Choices, an exploratory pilot program designed to demonstrate the feasibility of conducting dog walking as a component of a program focused on knowledge and awareness of nutrition and physical exercise in school-age children. A secondary purpose was identification of potential research questions arising from such a program.

Kids and K-9s for healthy choices program description

The program utilized didactic nutrition and physical activity education and demonstrations, guest speakers, human-animal interactions, and encouragement to engage in dog walking. The mission of the program was to provide a fun and educational program to heighten children's awareness of healthy food choices, promote regular exercise, increase self-esteem, and foster responsibilities within a community and family. The program founder (co-author Wright) wanted to provide a local program to which physicians could refer families with children who were overweight or at risk for overweight. The program consisted of two components, each called "projects." The shelter-based project served as the pilot for recruiting and exploring the feasibility of including human-dog interaction in health education. The school-based project served as the pilot for exploring the feasibility and children's acceptance of receiving health and fitness-related teaching in an afterschool format.

Shelter-based project

Participants

The shelter-based project targeted overweight and obese adolescents living in central Florida. Participants were recruited through the Children's Medical Services (CMS) Ocala area office. International Classification of Disease (ICD-9) codes were used to classify potential participants as overweight or obese. Children ages 13 through 16 with an obesity ICD-9 code (278.00-278.10) or a diabetic ICD-9 code (250.0-250.80) who were enrolled in CMS were contacted about participation. Parent and physician approvals were obtained for five middle school students who were subsequently enrolled in the shelter-based project.

Detailed project description

The shelter-based project served as the pilot for exploring the feasibility of including human-dog interaction in health education with overweight and obese adolescents at a local animal shelter. The participants and their families adopted a dog from the Humane Society or a local animal shelter and were asked to adhere to the following dog walking requirements for the duration of the eight-month project: to walk their dog for 30 minutes twice a day, one time being accompanied by a family member. Participants were given step-counting pedometers to track the distance of these walks (one mile= 2,000 steps).

The participants and their parents also attended one-hour long, bi-monthly meetings held on Saturdays at the Humane Society from April 2008 until November 2008. Each of these 16 sessions consisted of a nutrition and physical activity lesson, a dog lesson (proper care, grooming, or training), a planned physical activity (such as jump rope, Zumba dance, or walking with the shelter dogs), and a healthy food demonstration (a healthy recipe corresponding to the food group taught that lesson). Each of these sessions was conducted by volunteer registered nurses and social service specialists. Half of the sessions included guest speakers such as veterinarians, dog trainers, pediatricians, psychologists, and nutritionists who spoke about their particular area of expertise. The first six sessions were preceded by a mandatory dog obedience class also held at the Humane Society. Nine of the sessions included a lesson on self esteem and family unity, given by a child psychologist. During these lessons the participants wrote in a journal and talked about their feelings toward their family and friends.

Parents were also included in these lessons, and in addition, they received lessons on healthy cooking methods, how to shop on a budget, and how to address healthy choices as a family. The didactic teaching was aimed at making healthy choices and how those choices affect the child's and family's lifestyle.

Procedure

Prior to the beginning of the project, participants submitted parent authorized permission forms, a physician permission form, and a multimedia permission form. To track attendance for the shelter-based project, participants and their families were required to sign in at every meeting. Participants had their height and weight measured every fourth session by volunteer nurses. Their BMIs and BMI-for-age-and-sex percentiles were calculated using the CDC's Child and Teen BMI Calculator using information on their height, weight, gender, and date of birth (Figure 10.1). Participants were responsible for completing and returning monthly walking logs, used to track the date, pedometer steps, and accompaniment of their required dog walking sessions. To increase awareness of their current food choices, participants completed daily food logs for the seventh and eighth weeks of the project. In addition, the Humane Society administered compatibility tests to help each family determine suitable dog breeds that were a good match with their specific lifestyles and personalities.

Findings

The shelter-based project enrolled five participants: ages eleven to thirteen; three females, two males; four African Americans, one Caucasian; all five enrolled in Medicaid; one classified as overweight, four classified as obese. Project participation was inconsistent, with attendance dropping particularly in the summer months. All of the participants and their families adopted a dog within the first four months of the project.

Three participants reported their activity level prior to participation in the program as sedentary (less than 30 minutes of exercise per day), and two participants reported their prior activity level as moderate (moderate aerobic and/or strength training exercise 30 to 60 minutes on most days of the week). Upon the conclusion of the program, all participants reported their activity

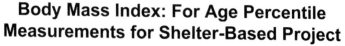

Figure 10.1. Shelter-based project participants' BMI-for-age-and-sex percentile measurements taken at the beginning and the end of the project.

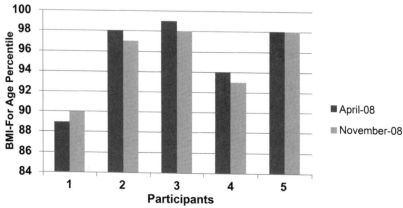

level as moderate or vigorous (moderate and vigorous activity 60 minutes every day of the week). A total of 513.76 miles were walked over eight months and an average of 13.45 miles per month was walked by each participant (based on their pedometer readings and walking log records). Over the course of the project, three participants' BMI-for-age-and-sex percentile measurements decreased by one percentile, one participant's percentile stayed the same, and one participant's percentile increased by one percentile. All but one participant decreased BMI measurements; the heaviest participant lost 15 pounds.

There was anecdotal evidence of the project's success, particularly the stories of Allison and Kevin (given pseudonyms to protect anonymity). Allison, a 12-year-old female with a sedentary lifestyle, started the shelter-based project with a BMI of 37 (which placed her in the 99th BMI- for-age-and-sex percentile). Allison received excellent grades in school, but she stated on the first day of the program that she had no friends and she "hated going to school" because she was picked on and teased. She reported no leisure or extracurricular activities, instead preferring to stay at home with her younger brother. Allison, her brother, and her mother were dedicated to the project and completed the food and walking logs in their entirety. Allison's family was looking for a small dog for which care would be easy. They looked for a number of weeks at the Humane Society dogs, but did not find the right one for them. One Saturday there was a notice at the Humane Society about a

10-pound Yorkshire terrier named Buddy that was in need of rescue at a location 30 minutes away. Allison and her mother drove to see the dog and instantly fell in love with Buddy, who quickly became Allison's constant companion. Allison stated at the end of the program that, "Now I have a reason to get up in the morning and go to school because I get to come home to Buddy!" Allison began to walk more and pay attention to what she ate. She went to dog obedience lessons and learned how to care for her new best friend. At the end of the eight-month program, Alison's BMI was 34.6 (down from 37), and she had walked 101 miles.

Kevin, a 13-year-old male, played some basketball at school, but he was very shy and had a BMI of 31 (which placed him in the obese category and in the 95th age percentile of BMI-for-age-and-sex). He came from a very large family; both he and his sister were adopted. Kevin's sister was highly allergic to animal dander so they were looking to adopt a dog that had hypoallergenic qualities. It took four months to find the right dog, but eventually they found Cody, an unidentified mixed breed, and adopted him from the animal shelter. While he was waiting to adopt this new best friend, Kevin attended project sessions with his mother and sister. After the dog adoption they walked the family dog regularly and participated fully in the project's activities. One day Kevin's mother called and said that he had been involved in an incident at school and would not be able to attend that week's session. He had been beaten in the boys' restroom. Kevin was a dedicated participant, however, after his incident, he began to walk even more, became more conscious of what he ate, and reported feeling better about himself. He gained self-confidence through his improved health and through project-related relationships with other participants and his dog. Kevin smiled when he spoke about the things he was teaching Cody and the great time they were having together. At the end of the program, Kevin's BMI was 29.3 (down from 31), and he had walked a total of 61 miles.

School-based project

Participants

The school-based project was aimed at central Florida elementary students enrolled in kindergarten through 5th grade. Letters of invitation to host the project were submitted to local private and public schools that operated after-school programs. A public magnet school responded with interest and agreed to add "Kids and K-9s" as an afterschool program option for their second and third grade students. Parent and physician waivers were obtained, and twenty students were subsequently enrolled in the fall 2009 semester and nine students were enrolled in the spring 2010 semester.

Detailed project description

The school-based project served as the pilot for exploring the feasibility and children's acceptance of receiving health and fitness-related teaching in an afterschool format at an elementary school. The overall goal was to increase nutrition and physical activity awareness and knowledge. The project consisted of two series of 14 weekly, one-hour long, afterschool sessions held on Tuesdays at a public magnet school in central Florida during the fall 2009 and the spring 2010 semesters. Each semester had the same 14 lessons, but different participants and guest speakers. Each of the 14 sessions included a nutrition and physical activity lesson, a dog lesson (proper care, grooming, or training), a planned physical activity, and highlighted a healthy food recipe (corresponding to the food group taught in that lesson). Five of the sessions also featured guest speakers such as a child psychologist who talked about self-esteem and the importance of expressing emotions. To increase activity levels, participants were encouraged to walk at least 15 minutes every day at home with their dogs or family members. The project used registered nurses and social service specialists as volunteers to supplement the on-site physical education teacher provided by the school to conduct these weekly sessions.

The fall semester group did not have any human-dog interactions in the classroom because the school would not allow the program to bring dogs on campus without an insurance policy. Kids and K-9s procured a policy in the spring of 2010, which led to an additional three guest speakers: dog trainers and handlers who were accompanied with their dogs during those sessions.

Procedure

Prior to the beginning of the project, participants submitted parent authorized permission forms, a physician permission form, and a multimedia permission form. We used parent demographic data collection questionnaires, walking logs to track activity levels, and pre- and post-project surveys containing a wide range of health questions, such as weekly eating, sleeping, and physical activity habits. The responses on frequency, length, and accompaniment of family members during dog walking were derived from self-reporting pre- and post-surveys and were only collected for those participants who owned a dog (n=12). The height and weight of each participant was measured monthly by the volunteer nurses and used to calculate their BMI.

Findings

The fall 2009 school-based project originally enrolled 20 students, however, only 17 students completed the project. The school would not permit dogs on campus without an insurance policy held by Kids and K-9s, and the lack of human-dog interactions was cited as the reason for dropping the project by the three participants who did so. The participants who completed the project were ages seven through nine; seven males and ten females; thirteen Caucasians, one African American, three Hispanic/Latinos; twelve owned at least one dog, five did not have access to a dog at home. Project attendance was consistent. All participants returned their pre- and post-surveys, walking logs, and parent demographic forms. The school helped arrange for healthy snacks at every session, welcomed guest speakers, and provided a central location for all of the volunteers, participants, and guest speakers to meet.

The average BMI of the fall 2009 semester group participants who had a dog was 16.4 (62nd BMI-for-age-and-sex percentile for boys and in the 59th BMI-for-age-and-sex percentile for girls). The average BMI of participants without a dog was 18.5 (88th BMI-for-age-and-sex percentile for boys and in the 85th BMI-for–age-and-sex percentile for girls). The twelve participants who owned a dog in the fall 2009 semester group were asked to track the frequency and duration of dog walking sessions and whether or not they were alone or accompanied by a family member or friend over the course of the project. The average frequency of all participant dog walking sessions was 0.92 times per week at the beginning of the project and 2.4 times per week at the end of the project. The average duration of participant dog walking sessions was 3.75 minutes at the beginning of the project and 13.75 minutes at the end of the project. The average times per week participants walked their dog with a family member or friend at the beginning of the project was 0.92; at the end of the project, the average was 2.25 times per week (Figure 10.2).

The spring 2010 school-based project enrolled nine students, but only eight students completed the project: ages seven through nine; two males and seven females; six Caucasians and two Hispanic/Latinos; four owned at least one dog and four did not. The one participant who left the project decided to attend another afterschool program offered by the school. The attendance of the remaining participants was consistent, and the school remained accommodating to the project. All of the spring 2010 semester participants returned their pre-surveys and parent demographic forms, however, only one participant returned their post-survey.

Because Kids and K-9s had an insurance policy by the start of the spring 2010 semester, dogs were permitted on campus, and the difference of hav-

Figure 10.2. Dog walking log information for school-based project, fall 2009 semester group participants.

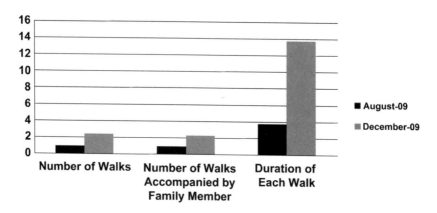

ing the dogs present at the sessions was immediately apparent. The enthusiasm of the children was overflowing. They were able to see the importance of nutrition and physical activity—side-by-side with what the dog needed and what they needed. Their questions were inexhaustible about animal behavior and what things the dogs liked and did not like to eat and do. One example of how the dog guest speakers affected the children was when a service dog visited the group. The dog and his owner showed the participants an animal food pyramid next to the human food pyramid and also demonstrated what tasks the service dog did to help its owner. The next day a grandparent of one of the participants remarked: "I just had to tell you that my granddaughter came home from your class yesterday and said that she was going to teach her dog to do the things she saw in class, that she had to take the dog for a walk every morning before school, and that we—as a family—had to be mindful of what we fed the dog."

Discussion

The overall content of the program (including both the shelter and the school-based projects) and the human-dog interactions received positive reviews from the participants and their families; all of the participants were attentive, participated in their respective project's activities, and got along well with each other. The participants who wore pedometers enjoyed using them to track their dog walking activities. Guest speakers were recruited from the local area and none indicated that transportation or location were a problem. In the shelter-based project, space, time, and monetary considerations had to be accounted for when selecting the appropriate dog for each family, a process that took up to four months and guidance from the Humane Society. Future Kids and K-9s projects will likely not stipulate the adoption of a dog as a program requirement. Although dog ownership was not reported as a burden by the participants, it is not realistic to assume that all future participants' families will be able to accommodate such a request. Further, selection bias would be problematic in future research studies on dog ownership with relation to healthy behavior modifications because only those who could afford a dog would be allowed to participate. Sustainability of the Kids and K-9s program and future similar projects will require further funding, volunteers, and participants.

The comprehensive educational components of the shelter-based project appeared to be enhanced by the human-animal interaction provided by the adoption of a dog and the regular walking of that dog. Because all of the participants were overweight or obese (according to their BMI-for-age-and-sex percentiles), physical activity through dog walking was an important focus of this project. The motivation provided by dogs was a qualitatively important factor in modifying the healthy lifestyle behaviors and choices of the program's participants. Although four of the five participants decreased their overall BMI measurements during the course of the project, their BMI-for-age-and-sex percentiles did not change significantly. No conclusions can be drawn because we were not conducting a controlled study. Further, extreme weight loss was not the goal of the program and therefore we did not expect to see significant decreases in BMI-for-age-and-sex percentiles in the short-term. However, the decreases in BMI for participants did represent some weight loss and participants reported feeling better about themselves at the end of the project. One participant had an increase in BMI and BMI-for-age-and-sex percentile. This adolescent did not attend six of the sixteen sessions.

Future projects of Kids and K-9s should focus less on physical health measures such as BMI and more on other factors that have been reported to positively affect healthy behaviors. Little is known about the outcomes of BMI measurement programs, including the relationship with weight-related knowledge, attitudes, and behaviors of youth and their families (Nihiser et al., 2007). There are no clear data to suggest that tracking and reporting BMI measurements to students and parents translates into modification of healthy behaviors (Evansa & Sonnevillea, 2009). In addition, including BMI screening and measurements in adolescent health projects may have consequences that are not yet fully understood, such as weight-related teasing, stigmatization, and eating disorder risks (Evansa & Sonnevillea, 2009).

The shelter-based project format was not ideal. All of the parents noted that consistent transportation and attendance was a hardship because the sessions were held on Saturdays, they were required to attend with their children, and the Humane Society was not in a central location. Additional barriers to participation were hot weather and vacation time taken during the summer months of the project. Location is important for participation. Future projects would likely be more successful operating in a location where children are already gathered. Failing that option, transportation should be provided.

In the school-based project, the participants were already on-site, requiring no additional transportation from their parents or the school, resulting in consistent attendance in weekly sessions. The afterschool format of the project provided a fun addition to the school day for students who were already focused on learning. The project lost participants to other afterschool programs offered by the school, especially in the spring 2010 semester when more fine arts programs became available to students. In addition, enrollment was lower in the spring 2010 group because classroom human-dog interactions were not advertised; the insurance policy was not acquired until after participants were enrolled. The need for marketing the program became readily apparent. The spring 2010 project group encountered difficulty in obtaining completed post-project surveys. These documents were given to the students at the last session, which occurred during the last week of the school semester. Students did not have an opportunity to return the surveys after receiving them in the session and taking them home to complete with the help of their parents. The fall 2009 semester group were also given their post-surveys during the last session in December, but had the opportunity to return the surveys in January when they returned to school. Future projects should either design the survey to be completed by the participants during a session or distribute the post-surveys to the participants during the second-to-last session, allowing ample time to complete and return the surveys by the last session.

Investigators have shown the effectiveness of school-based health interventions: multi-component interventions aimed at adolescents have shown success in preventing weight gain (Singh, Chin A Paw, Brug, & Van Mechelen, 2007) and in increasing health knowledge and certain dietary behaviors (Harrell, Davy, Stewart, & King, 2005). Afterschool settings in particular have been attracting attention because they allow access to a large number of children and provide a unique opportunity for the implementation of multi-component programs involving nutrition, physical activity, and parents (Kelder, Hoelscher, Barroso, Walker, Cribb, & Hu, 2005). The afterschool time period is one of the largest blocks of discretionary time in a child's typical day and may represent a potential avenue to provide opportunities for increasing physical activity (Kaplah, Liverman, & Kraak, 2004).

A literature review of interventions to promote physical activity in children and adolescents reported strong evidence for the effectiveness of school-based interventions including family or community involvement, multi-component interventions, and educational interventions with policy and environmental changes (Van Sluijs, McMinn, & Griffin, 2007). The Kids and K-9s programs demonstrated the feasibility of a school-based intervention with an educational focus; however, future projects should consider incorporating other strategies such as policy and environmental modifications in order to see the greatest and most long-lasting effects on participants.

The CDC recommends the following strategies for operating a successful school health program: working with the school to adopt a formal nutrition policy (including food services), establishing a sequential and comprehensive curriculum, and involving student's families and the community (CDC, 1996). The Child and Adolescent Trial for Cardiovascular Health (CATCH), a NIH-funded project testing the effectiveness of an intervention for third- to fifth-grade students (in 96 schools nationally) targeting healthy eating habits, increased physical activity and a non-smoking lifestyle. The investigators suggested that teacher training was an important factor in achieving sustainability of a school-based health education program (Hoelscher et al., 2004). Strengthening and expanding relationships with host schools could help to sustain and improve feasibility of the Kids and K-9s program. While we experienced excellent support, this is an important factor to consider in developing such programs.

The increase in family member/friend accompaniment found in our projects raises potential research questions about the effect of companions on motivation to exercise. Social support, such as family and peer influences, has been related to physical activity in children (Taylor, Baranowski, & Sallis, 1994). Family support is important for encouraging children to be physical active (Brockman, Jago, Fox, Thompson, Cartwright, & Page, 2010). Although schools have traditionally provided and promoted physical activity directly, through physical education curricula and afterschool intramural sports, there has been recent interest in exploring the potential of collaboration between schools and community-based programs to increase the physical activity levels of students (Pate, Davis, Robinson, Stone, McKenzie, & Young, 2006). The Kids and K-9s school-based project is a testament to the feasibility of such a collaboration, however, research is required to fully understand the efficacy of specific formats and project components. Given the anectdotal observations of our program and the established impacts of dog ownership and dog walking on health, the efficacy of dog walking as a compent of a health education program should be studied.

Incorporating human-dog interactions and stronger partnerships with host schools with an afterschool project format may be the ideal approach of future Kids and K-9s programs. Through our preliminary efforts, we learned that the school-based approach was the most logistically practical one. The children were receptive to the school-based format, and we learned that it was possible to facilitate dog walking and human-dog interactions through such a program. However, research is needed to test the efficacy of such projects in delivering standardized health education information and encouraging children to exercise through dog walking. Issues arising in the projects, such as the reliability of the participants' self reports of exercise, intervention fidelity, and identification and systematic measurement of key outcome variables must be addressed in order for such programs to effectively generate evidence that can inform others interested in implementing programs involving dog walking for children.

Conclusion

Our projects showed that a school-based program involving dog walking is logistically possible and may represent a unique approach to positively impacting the health and well-being of children and families by facilitating healthy lifestyle choices. Pets play a large role in American family culture and in daily activities. According to the 2009-2010 National Pet Owners' Survey, Americans own 77.5 million dogs and 39% of households own at least one dog (Humane Society, 2010). A review of relevant literature presents a strong case that dogs provide a number of health benefits to humans. Encouraging overweight or at-risk for overweight adolescents and their families to adopt dog walking as a source of fun and healthy physical activity, may have implications for our nation's physical, mental, and social health.

Incorporating man's best friend into everyday healthy activities may motivate children and families and encourage their continued well-being. An exercise class may last only 10 to 12 weeks, diets get boring, but one's dog is always there, ready to give love and ready for a walk or other engaging interaction. In the process of expansion and further development, Kids and K-9s for Healthy Choices will focus on helping children establish long-lasting habits of making healthy food choices, increasing regular physical activity, strengthening family bonds, and most importantly, fostering the relationship of love and respect between dogs and humans that allow the aforementioned benefits to blossom. Have you walked your dog today?

Acknowledgments

Kids and K-9s is supported with grant money from the Robert Wood Johnson Foundation Executive Nurse Fellowship program, the State of Florida Department of Health Children's Medical Service Ocala area office, and donations from central Florida corporations and individuals. Iams™ donated the pedometers used by the shelter-based project, as well as water bottles, dog leashes, dog food coupons, and dog bandanas.

Kids and K-9s would like to especially thank Debra Grant, Linda Beckwith, Abigail Smith, and all of the volunteers and guest speakers who have donated their time and their talents.

References

American Academy of Child & Adolescent Psychiatry. (2008). Pets and children: Facts for families. Retrieved from http://www.aacap.org/cs/root/facts_for_families/pets_and_children

Anderson, W. P., Reid, C. M., & Jennings, G. L. (1992). Pet ownership and risk factors for cardiovascular disease. *Medical Journal of Australia, 157*(5), 298-301.

Bayer Diabetes Care. (2010). Information-motivation-behavior skills analysis advance understanding of barriers to self-monitoring of blood glucose. Bayer HealthCare AG. Retrieved from http://www.press.bayer.com/baynews/baynews.nsf/id/14B17A618708A115C125774D0034C971?Open&ccm=001

Brockman, R., Jago, R., Fox, K. R., Thompson, J. L., Cartwright, C., & Page, A. S. (2009). Get off the sofa and go and play: Family and socioeconomic influences on the physical activity of 10-11 year old children. *BMC Public Health, 9*, 253. Retrieved from http://www.medscape.com/viewarticle/713664

Centers for Disease Control and Prevention. (1996). Guidelines for school health programs to promote lifelong healthy eating. *Morbidity and Mortality Weekly Reports, 45*(RR-9), 1-33

Centers for Disease Control and Prevention. (2002). The importance of regular physical activity for children. Centers for Disease Control and Prevention.

Centers for Disease Control and Prevention. (2002). The benefits of physical activity. National Center for Chronic Disease Prevention and Health Promotion, Division of Adolescent and School Health. Retrieved from http://www.cdc.gov/youthcampaign/pressroom/article/physical.htm

Centers for Disease Control and Prevention. (2009). About BMI for children and teens. Retrieved from http://www.cdc.gov/healthyweight/assessing/bmi/childrens_BMI/about_childrens_BMI.html

Centers for Disease Control and Prevention. (2009). Overweight and obesity: Causes and consequences. Retrieved from http://www.cdc.gov/obesity/causes/index.html

Centers for Disease Control and Prevention. (2010). School health programs: Improving the health of our nation's youth, at a glance 2010. Retrieved from http://www.cdc.gov/chronicdisease/resources/publications/aag/dash.htm

Evansa, E. W., & Sonnevillea, K. R. (2009) BMI report cards: Will they pass or fail in the fight against pediatric obesity? *Current Opinion in Pediatrics, 21,* 431–436.

Fisher, J. D., Fisher, W. A., Bryan, A. D., & Misovich, S. J. (2002). Information-motivation-behavioral skills model-based HIV risk behavior change intervention for inner city high school youth. *Health Psychology, 21,* 177-186. Retrieved from http://digitalcommons.uconn.edu/cgi/viewcontent.cgi?article=1002&context=chip_docs

Fisher, J., & Fisher, W. (2002). The information-motivation-behavioral skills model. In R. Diclemente, R. Crosby, & M. Kegler (Eds.), *Emerging theories in health promotion practice and research* (pp. 40-70). San Francisco: Jossey-Bass.

Garrity, T. F., Stallones, L., Marx, M. B., & Johnson, T. P. (1989). Pet ownership and attachment as supportive factors in the health of the elderly. *Anthrozoos, 3*(1), 35-44.

Ham, S., & Epping, J. (2006). Dog walking and physical activity in the United States. *Preventing Chronic Disease,* 3(2) A47. Retrieved from http://www.ncbi.nlm.nih.gov/pmc/articles/PMC1563959

Harrell, T. K., Davy, B. M., Stewart, J. L, & King, D. S. (2005). Effectiveness of a school-based intervention to increase health knowledge of cardiovascular disease risk factors among rural Mississippi middle school children. *Southern Medical Journal, 98* (12), 1173-1180.

Hoelscher, D. M., Feldman, H. A., Johnson, C. C., Lytle, L. A., Osganian, S. K., Parcel, G. S., Kelder, S. H., Stone, E. J., & Nader, P. R. (2004). School-based health education programs can be maintained over time: Results from the CATCH institutionalization study. *Preventive Medicine, 38*(5), 594-606.

Humane Society of the United States. (2009). U.S. pet ownership statistics. Retrieved from http://www.humanesociety.org/issues/pet_overpopulation/facts/pet_ownership_statistics.html

Kaplah, J. P., Liverman, C. T., & Kraak, V.I. (Eds.), (2004). *Preventing childhood obesity: Health in the balance.* Institute of Medicine (US) Committee on Prevention of Obesity in Children and Youth. Washington, DC: Institute of Medicine, 237–284.

Katcher, A. H. (1982). Are companion animals good for your health? *Aging, Sept-Oct*, 331-332.

Kelder, S., Hoelscher, D. M., Barroso, C. S., Walker, J. L., Cribb, P., & Hu, S. (2005). The CATCH kids club: A pilot after-school study for improving elementary students' nutrition and physical activity. *Public Health Nutrition*, *8*(2), 133-140.

Kushner, R. F., Blanter, D. J., Jewell, D. E., & Rudloff, K. (2006). The PPET study: People and pets exercising together. *Obesity, 14*, 1762-1770. Retrieved from http://www.nature.com/oby/journal/v14/n10/full/oby2006203a.html

Lockwood, R. (1983). The influence of animals on social perception. In A. H. Katcher & A. M. Beck, (Eds.), *New perspectives on our lives with companion animals*. Philadelphia, PA: University of Pennsylvania Press.

Messent, P. R. (1983). Social facilitations of contact with other people by pet dogs. In A. H. Katcher & A. M. Beck, (Eds.), *New perspectives on our lives with companion animals*. Philadelphia, PA: University of Pennsylvania Press.

National Center for Chronic Disease Prevention and Health Promotion. (2010). School health programs: Improving the health of our nation's youth. U.S. Department of Health and Human Services and the Centers for Disease Control and Prevention. Retrieved from http://www.cdc.gov/chronicdisease/resources/publications/aag/pdf/2010/dash-2010.pdf

Nihiser, A. J., Lee, S. M., Wechsler, H., McKenna, M., Odom, E., Reinold, C., Thompson. D., & Grummer-Strawn, L. (2007). Body mass index measurement in schools. *Journal of School Health, 77*, 651-671.

Ogden, C., & Carroll, M. D. (2010). Prevalence of obesity among children and adolescents: United States, trends 1963-1965 through 2007-2008. Centers for Disease Control and Prevention. Retrieved from http://www.cdc.gov/nchs/data/hestat/obesity_child_07_08/obesity_child_07_08.pdf

Ogden, C., Carroll, M. D., & Flegal, K. M. (2008). High body mass index for age among US children and adolescents. *Journal of the American Medical Association*, *299*(20), 2401-2405.

Owen, C. G., Nightingale, C. M., Rudnicka, A. R., Ekelund, U., McMinn, A. M., Van Sluijs, E. M., & Whincup, P. H. (2010). Family dog ownership and levels of physical activity in childhood: Findings from the child heart and health study in England. *American Journal of Public Health*. DOI:10.2105/AJPH.2009.188193.

Pate, R. R., Davis, M. G., Robinson, T. N., Stone, E. J., McKenzie, T. L., & Young, J. C. (2006). Promoting physical activity in children and youth: A leadership role for schools. A scientific statement from the American Heart Association Council on Nutrition, Physical Activity, and Metabolism in collaboration with the Councils on Cardiovascular Disease in the Young. *Cardiovascular Nursing*, *114*, 1214-1224

Roberts, D., & Foehr, U. (2004). *Kids and media in America*. Cambridge, MA: Cambridge University Press.

Robert Wood Johnson Foundation and the American Heart Association. (2008). A nation at risk: Obesity in the United States. Retrieved from http://www.rwjf.org/files/publications/other/AH_NationAtRisk.pdf

Singh, A. S., Chin A., Paw, M. J. A., Brug, J., & Van Mechelen, W. (2007). Short-term effects of school-based weight gain prevention among adolescents. *Archives of Pediatric and Adolescent Medicine, 161,* 565-571.

Taylor, W. C., Baranowski, T., & Sallis, J. F. (1994) Family determinants of childhood physical activity: A social-cognitive model. Advances in Exercise Adherence. Champaign, Ill: Human Kinetics, 319-342.

United States Department of Health and Human Services. (2008). Physical activity guidelines for Americans: Chapter 3: Active children and adolescents. Retrieved from http://www.health.gov/paguidelines/guidelines/chapter3.aspx

Van Sluijs, E., McMinn, A. M., & Griffin, S. J. (2007) Effectiveness of interventions to promote physical activity in children and adolescents: Systematic review of controlled trials. Medical Research Council Epidemiology Unit, Institute of Metabolic Sciences, Addenbrooke's Hospital, Cambridge CB2 0QQ. DOI:10.1136/bmj.39320.843947.BE.

Whitaker, R. C., Wright, J. A., Pepe, M. S., Seidel, K. D., & Dietz, W. H. (1997). Predicting obesity in young adulthood from childhood and parental obesity. *New England Journal of Medicine, 37*(13), 869–873.

Chapter 11

Future directions in dog walking

Rebecca A. Johnson, Alan M. Beck, Sandra McCune, James A. Griffin, and Layla Esposito

The views expressed in this manuscript are those of the authors and do not necessarily represent those of the National Institutes of Health, *Eunice Kennedy Shriver* National Institute of Child Health and Human Development, or the U.S. Department of Health and Human Services and Mars, Incorporated.

The goal of this chapter is to synthesize what has been presented in the preceding chapters and to pose new directions for the dog walking field. After an overarching discussion of the benefits of dog walking, we challenge investigators to push research in this area to new heights, perhaps leading the rest of the human-animal interaction (HAI) field in similar directions.

Dog walking as purposeful and supportive physical activity

Physical activity (PA) has well documented benefits, but most of the world fails to meet recommended guidelines for PA (Bauman, chapter 3, this volume). Physical inactivity is not limited to wealthier developed nations, but increasingly is being recognized as a global epidemic (Guthold, Cowan, Autenrieth, Kann, & Riley 2010). In their study of PA and sedentary behavior among schoolchildren in a 34-country comparison across Africa, the Americas, Southeast Asia, the Western Pacific region, and the Eastern Mediterranean, Guthold and colleagues found very few students engaged in sufficient PA. This was a particular issue in girls; only 15% of girls and 24% of boys met national PA recommendations. The study concluded that immediate action is required worldwide to increase levels of PA among schoolchildren. Dog walking would seem to be an obvious means of increasing PA, but as was stated in Bauman's chapter, most dog owners do not walk their dogs. However, those dog owners who do walk their dogs are very likely to reach recommendations for PA (Wood & Christian, chapter 4, this volume).

A major motivator for walking as a form of PA is its accessibility. It is not technically difficult, does not require expensive equipment, and can be done almost anywhere and at any time by almost anybody. Dog walking is accessible for the same reasons but has the additional motivator of being "purposeful walking." "Dog obligation" is a strong motivator for many owners who accept that a daily walk is a reasonable expectation for a dog. The sense of responsibility to walk a dog daily is an important correlate of dog walking intention and behavior (Brown & Rhodes 2006; Cutt et al., 2008). This sense of purpose in walking the dog versus just walking alone or even with a human companion for a walk can be a powerful motivator.

Dogs also provide an emotional motivator for walking. Owners may be positively reinforced by their dogs when they take them for a walk or even look like they might. When an owner is attached to his or her dog, being able to do something so positive for that beloved family member is likely to be rewarding in and of itself, but can be especially so when reinforced by enthusiastic dog behavior. Dog walking is a great way to build the bond between owner and dog and, in turn, increase the motivation of the owner to meet the dog's need for walking.

Another form of emotional support arising from dog walking is the social facilitation effect of walking with a dog, which can increase the amount, quality, and frequency of social interaction between people meeting outside (McNicholas & Collis, 2000; Cutt et al., 2008; Messent, 1983). The resulting "social capital" can have far-reaching benefits for the residents involved in these interactions (Wood & Christian, chapter 4, this volume).

Unfortunately, dog obesity is now a parallel issue to human obesity. Hurley, Elliott, and Lund (chapter 8, this volume) reviewed risk factors for obesity in dogs including genetics, concurrent diseases, demographics, diet, and lifestyle, but also interestingly including attributes of the owner-dog relationship (Kienzle, Bergler, & Mandernach, 1998; Morris, Montoya, Bautista, Juste, Suarez, Peña, McCune, & Hackett, 2007; Courcier, 2009). Obesity is also becoming an associated issue between pets and owners; the association between overweight/obese parents and their children within households is now also seen between overweight/obese owners and their dogs within households (Monterio et al., 2004; Berkowitz et al., 2005; Epstein, 1998; Kienzle et al., 1998). While obesity is a health issue at all ages, obese children also experience stigmatization and bullying more than normal weight children (Lumeng et al., 2010). Dog walking is a good form of PA for both dogs and owners who need to redress the balance between PA and calories consumed.

Dogs may benefit in other ways from being walked. Walking should be a fun activity that is good for both the dog's and the owner's health, and not something that is done just because the dog must walk. In addition, walking the dog can help resolve dog problems including boredom and unwanted behaviors. Walking the dog twice a day for 30 to 60 minutes may help make the dog calmer and happier; excess energy is spent and the dog is usually mentally and emotionally stimulated by socializing with other dogs and people.

Dog walking and childhood obesity

The epidemic of childhood overweight and obesity affects approximately one out of three children in the United States (Ogden, Carroll, Curtin, Lamb, & Flegal, 2010) and is related to a host of physical and psychological consequences (e.g., type 2 diabetes, high blood pressure, dyslipidemia, social discrimination), which often continue into adulthood (Daniels, 2009). Unfortunately, efforts to prevent and treat childhood obesity on a population level have been largely ineffective or unsustainable, as evidenced by continuing and often worsening trends (e.g., Bethell, Simpson, Stumbo, Adam, & Gombojav, 2010). Although overweight and obesity primarily result from energy imbalance (calories consumed exceed calories expended), the problem can best be characterized as "a medical manifestation of the complex interplay of biology and social change" (Huang & Glass, 2008). Thus, understanding childhood obesity requires taking a complex systems approach, which considers the impact of multiple levels of socioecological risks, from individual level factors to macrosocial factors, on individual behavior (Huang & Glass, 2008).

Within this complex systems framework, it is important to consider which barriers and facilitators enable or constrain obesogenic behaviors (Glass & McAtee, 2006), including physical inactivity. Increasing the number of opportunities for PA for children (in combination with improved quality of diet) is clearly part of the solution to curbing the epidemic. Dog walking is a great example of providing one such opportunity for children and families.

Dog walking can be beneficial to maintaining energy balance in children. It has been estimated that the average energy gap for children (daily imbalance of calories consumed to calories expended resulting in overweight) ranges from 46 to 72 kilocalories per day to 110 to 165 kilocalories per day (Plachta-Danielzik, Landsberg, Bosy-Westphal, Johannsen, Lange, & Müller, 2008; Wang, Gortmaker, Sobol, & Kuntz, 2006). The addition of a daily routine of dog walking could contribute to reducing or even eliminating this gap. Because parents are the most influential role models for their children, activities that all family members can participate in should be encouraged. Regular dog walking provides an opportunity for the family to engage in a more active lifestyle, while parents are modeling the behavior for their children to learn from and eventually participate in independently. Parents should also be encouraged to emphasize the importance of PA for the health of the family dog, and teach caretaking behaviors (e.g., feeding, grooming) to gradually provide the child with a sense of responsibility for the dog's well-being.

At present, there is a paucity of research examining the impact of dog walking on child health and weight status, and a number of different types of research are needed. First, nationally representative surveillance data are necessary to determine the prevalence of dog ownership and the frequency of dog walking among owners and their children. Second, the majority of studies of dog walking (predominantly in adults) rely on cross-sectional designs, preventing the exploration of causality or the temporal relationships among variables of interest. Thus, there is a critical need for longitudinal cohort studies to determine the impact of dog walking on weight status and health. Finally, although difficult to design, the field is lacking randomized controlled trials of pet ownership and health.

Dog walking across cultures

The relatively rapid growth of research into dog walking as a sub-discipline of HAI may speak to the versatility of this activity across populations and settings. Given the ease of walking a dog for exercise (it can presumably be done anywhere without cost beyond expenses associated with keeping a dog, can be altered to suit the athletic ability of the person, and demands minimal gear to accomplish), a logical conclusion would be that everyone who owns a dog would walk it for physical activity. Two of the papers in this volume show readers that this is not always the case (Thorpe et al.; Bauman et al.). In fact there may be differences in populations or their circumstances that may make dog walking less appealing or possible. For example, in one of the few studies conducted to date with a non-Caucasian sample, older Latinos in the United States were found to be very strongly bonded with their dogs but did not necessarily exercise with them (Johnson & Meadows, 2002). Epidemiological data compiled by Bauman and colleagues in this volume show that while the prevalence of dog-keeping in industrialized countries is quite high, across studies, dog owners do not necessarily meet recommended daily PA levels.

Ethnic and socioeconomic differences may help to explain the fact that owning a dog does not necessarily equate with walking a dog. In the Wood and Christian chapter, the authors demonstrate that dog walking may contribute to positive perceptions about one's neighborhood. The notion of dog walking contributing to social capital is an appealing one, but may be bound to middle or upper socioeconomic status. Annual costs of keeping a dog may preclude pet ownership for large segments of the population. However, even for those who can afford to own a dog, if a neighborhood is unsafe or perceived to be unsafe, dog walking may have no impact on social capital because it may be dangerous to walk a dog. This may especially be the case if free-range dogs are perceived as dangerous; people may be less likely to walk their own dogs. The reality is that true stray or free-ranging dogs account for a small portion of the dog bite problem, which is caused by loose owned dogs (Beck, 1985, 1991, 2002). However, if dogs are kept as sources of protection, then walking them takes them away from the home that they are protecting, and may be unlikely. There is also some evidence that walking dogs around natural settings may reduce the possibility of seeing wildlife; walkers may want to enjoy those areas without their dogs (Banks & Bryant, 2007; Sterl & Brandenburg, 2008). In addition, pet keeping practices in rural areas where dogs regularly have more outdoor time may not include formal dog walking; both owner and dog may actually gain more exercise but may not report this as "dog walking."

Beyond the conjecture, little is known about dog walking in ethnically and socioeconomically diverse populations because there has been little study in this area. In one study, Japanese older adults were found to receive cardiovascular benefits from dog walking (Motooka, Koike, Yokoyama, & Kennedy, 2006), but further study is needed of diverse populations. Researchers do not yet know the "boundaries" of dog walking across cultures, nor do they know how cultural beliefs about dogs may affect dog walking patterns.

Methodological issues and dog walking research

A central question addressed by this volume is how well dog walking studies can withstand scientific scrutiny. On one hand, there is a body of research findings documenting the beneficial effects that dog walking can bestow on both the dog and his or her owner (Johnson & McKenney, this volume; Bauman, Christian, Thorpe, & Macniven, this volume). On the other hand, many of these studies are characterized by methodological and conceptual weaknesses that limit the interpretation of their findings (Johnson, 2010). What will it take to advance the evidence base in this area?

The first discussion of this issue appeared in a peer-reviewed medical journal 26 years ago (Beck & Katcher, 1984). The issue is periodically revived, and recently authors have questioned why more research has not been conducted in the HAI field in general. Griffin, McCune, Maholmes, and Hurley (2010a) have noted the need for increased methodological rigor and the use of sophisticated research designs (Kazdin, 2010), and they have offered directions for future HAI research (Griffin, McCune, Maholmes, & Hurley, 2010b). There are several research designs and methodology issues that the next generation of dog walking studies will need to address if this line of research is to move to the next level of scientific rigor.

A primary reason empirical knowledge on the benefits of dog walking has not accumulated more quickly relative to the number of studies conducted is the inherent difficulty associated with studying the phenomena. For example, the most straightforward way to study the effects of dog walking on a child's overall health and well-being would be to randomly assign children at birth to grow up with a dog, a fish, or no pet at all, and to monitor both their physical activity level and weight management with the "dog" and "fish" groups relative to children in the "no pet" control group. Of course, one could never ethically conduct such a study, so researchers are limited to using survey data to study children who do or do not have pets for a variety of reasons, knowing that these children and their families may systematically differ on a number of important variables that affect a child's health and activity level, but may have nothing to do with pet ownership and dog walking per se (e.g., income level, parent's health). There are statistical techniques (e.g., propensity score matching) available to help control for these differences in large longitudinal survey databases, but it is still possible that unmeasured variables are actually responsible for any between group differences that would otherwise be attributed to dog walking.

On the other end of the age spectrum, multiple studies documented in this volume have been conducted that randomly assign older adults to dog walking, buddy walking, or no treatment control groups. However, even this approach has its limitations. Clearly seniors with dog phobias or allergies would be less likely to agree to participate, and those who desire to be in the dog walking group may be unwilling to risk the chance that they would be randomly assigned to the no treatment control group. However, these issues can be dealt with by assessing history of dog ownership, animal phobias, and allergy issues prior to randomization, and making it clear that all study participants will be able to participate in the dog walking group once the study is over.

Once a volunteer subject pool is established, there are design and measurement issues that further complicate how to conduct a dog walking study. The most obvious is that the study participants will know whether or not they have been assigned to the dog walking group. This makes it impossible to tell if the presence of the dog is having an effect on the health outcomes or if it is just the novelty of having a dog to walk with or the desire to produce a positive research outcome that results in differences from the control group. The inability to conduct "blind" research, where the subject, and sometimes the researchers themselves, do not know if the subject is receiving the treatment or a placebo (e.g., a sugar pill) is an inherent limitation of HAI efficacy research, just as it is with other behavioral intervention research. Although it is possible to have alternate treatment conditions (e.g., a human rather than a canine walking buddy), such designs require a larger subject pool and still do not completely rule out the possibility of spurious results.

Once a study design has been established, the researchers also must decide which measures will be used to capture both what takes place during the dog walking activity and the health outcomes they hope to achieve for the senior participants. Unfortunately, at this stage of the study, many HAI researchers decide to create their own measures, either because they have not reviewed the literature on similar studies and the measures that have been used, or because their search of the literature did not reveal any measures that they felt captured what they want to measure in their study. It is difficult to compare results across studies if the same or comparable measures are not used. Most researcher-developed measures lack information on their psychometric properties (i.e., reliability and validity), making it difficult to know if two different measures of the same outcome (e.g., activity level) are measuring the same thing and would produce the same results if used simultaneously with the same subject. Of course, there are times when researchers have no option other than creating their own measures. However, the use of some standard measures (in addition to the researcher-developed measures), such as accelerometers and other direct measures of human and canine activity level, coupled with standard measures of health outcomes (e.g., Body Mass Index [BMI], blood pressure, and serum cholesterol) would allow both the direct comparison of outcomes across studies and meta-analytic studies to detect patterns of outcomes that might be difficult to detect with a single study.

The research examples above only touch on the design, methodology, and data analytic issues that must be addressed in order to increase the rigor and utility of dog walking research. A great deal more can and has been said about research design, methodology, and analytic approaches; reviews of other types of HAI interventions (Marino & Lilienfeld, 2007) should be referenced to understand why insufficient attention to these factors limits the conclusions that can be drawn from a given study. As evidenced by this volume, dog walking researchers have persisted despite the difficulties inherent in conducting research in this field, and they have made significant progress in advancing our understanding of how we can harness the power of the human-canine bond to address public health issues such as obesity and sedentary lifestyle.

Research questions for future dog walking studies

Many additional research questions need to be answered to move forward the field of HAI, and specifically dog walking. For example, not all dog owners walk their dogs regularly, so it will be important to understand if there are unique characteristics of families or the elderly who walk their dog versus those who do not. How might these characteristics mediate or moderate the relationship between dog walking and weight? There may be associations between dog walking and other health-related behaviors that influence weight status. What are the barriers and facilitators of dog walking in specific populations such as children and senior citizens (e.g., neighborhood safety, walkable streets, open spaces, ability to control the dog), and how can interventions increase the likelihood of overcoming these concerns? Does educating children, parents, and the elderly about the importance of PA for pet health increase their motivation to walk the dog or translate into engagement in other forms of PA? We also need to know what is the optimal duration and intensity of dog walking for children and older adults, or even playing with the dog, to gain a beneficial effect. Finally, researchers should focus on the development and dissemination of family- and community-based intervention programs that promote dog walking, such as the "Walk a Hound, Lose a Pound" program, described in chapter 6 of this volume.

The rapid growth of interest in dog walking research

One important lesson learned from the papers presented in this volume is just how quickly a phenomenon can catch on in academic circles and grow into its own movement within a field. In 2006, a dog walking research interest group formed with two members. At writing of this volume, the group consisted of over 50 members worldwide who either conduct dog walking research or have a strong interest in the subject. Dubbed the "International Dog-Walking Activity Group" (ID-WAG), the group provides a collaborative network to propel forward the dog walking field.

Perhaps the rapid growth of this field will make dog walking a viable option as a community intervention to facilitate healthy behavior across populations. As this growth occurs, we hope that strong scientific inquiry will grow accordingly.

References

Anonymous. (1999). Neighborhood safety and the prevalence of physical inactivity—selected states, 1996. MMWR. Morbidity and Mortality Weekly Report. Atlanta: Feb 26, 48(7), 143-146.

Anonymous. (2007). Dog walking scares away the local wildlife. *New Scientist*, 195(2620), 6.

Banks, P. B., & Bryant, J.V. (2007). Four-legged friend or foe? Dog walking displaces native birds from natural areas. *Biology Letters*, *3*(6), 611-613.

Beck, A. M. (1991). The epidemiology and prevention of animal bites. *Seminars in Veterinary Medicine and Surgery (Small Animal)*, *6*(3), 186-191.

Beck, A. M. (2002). *The ecology of stray dogs: A study of free-ranging urban animals.* West Lafayette, IN: Purdue University Press.

Beck, A. M., & Jones, B. (1985). Unreported dog bites in children. *Public Health Reports*, *100*, 315-321.

Beck, A. M, & Katcher, A .H. (1984). A new look at pet-facilitated therapy. *Journal of the American Veterinary Medical Association*, *184*, 414-421.

Berkowitz, R. I., et al. (2005) Growth of children at high risk of obesity during the first 6 years of life: Implications for prevention *Am J Clin Nutr*, *81*, 140-146

Bethell, C., Simpson, L., Stumbo, S., Carle, A., & Gombojav, N. (2010). National, state and local disparities in childhood obesity. *Health Affairs*, *29*, 347-356.

Brown, S. G., & Rhodes, R. E. (2006). Relationships among dog ownership and leisure-time walking in western Canadian adults. *American Journal of Preventive Medicine*, *30*(2), 131-136.

Courcier, E. A. (2009). Canine obesity: Do owners see what you see? Proceedings of BSAVA Congress.

Cutt, H., Giles-Corti, B., & Knuiman, M. (2008). Encouraging physical activity through dog walking: Why don't some owners walk with their dog? *Preventive Medicine*, *46*(2), 120-126.

Daniels, S. R. (2009). Complications of obesity in children and adolescents. *International Journal of Obesity*, *33*(Supplement 1), S60-S65.

Epstein, L. (1996) A family-based intervention program for obese childen. *International Journal of Obesity*, *20*, S14-S21.

Glass, T. A., & McAtee, M. J. (2006). Behavioral science at the crossroads in public health: Extending horizons, envisioning the future. Social *Science and Medicine, 62*, 1650-1671.

Griffin, J. A., McCune, S., Maholmes, V., & Hurley, K. (2010a). Introduction to human-animal interaction research. In P. McCardle, S. McCune, J. A. Griffin, & V. Maholmes (Eds.), *How animals affect us: Examining the influence of human-animal interaction on child development and human health* (pp. 3-9). Washington, DC: American Psychological Association Press.

Griffin, J. A., McCune, S., Maholmes, V., & Hurley, K. (2010b). Scientific research on human-animal interaction: A framework for future studies. In P. McCardle, S. McCune, , J. A. Griffin, L. Esposito, & L. S. Freund (Eds.), *Animals in our lives: Human-animal interaction in family, community & therapeutic settings* (pp. 227-236). Baltimore, MD: Brookes Publishing.

Guthold, R., Cowan, M. J., Autenrieth, C. S., Kann, L., & Riley, L. M. (2010). Physical activity and sedentary behavior among schoolchildren: A 34 country comparison. *The Journal of Pediatrics, 157*(1), 43-49.

Huang, T. K., & Glass, T. A. (2008). Transforming research strategies for understanding and preventing obesity. *Journal of the American Medical Association, 300*, 1811-1813.

Johnson, R. A. (2010). Health benefits of animal-assisted intervention. In P. McCardle, S. McCune, J. A. Griffin, & V. Maholmes (Eds.), *How animals affect us: Examining the influence of human-animal interaction on child development and human health* (pp.183-192). Washington, DC: American Psychological Association Press.

Johnson, R. A., & Meadows, R. L. (2002). Older Latinos, pets and health. *Western Journal of Nursing Research, 24*(6), 609-620.

Johnson, R. A., & Meadows, R L. (2010). Dog walking: Motivation for adherence to a walking program. *Clinical Nursing Research, 19*(4) 387–402.

Kazdin, A. (2010). Establishing the effectiveness of animal-assisted therapies: What types of research designs and findings would build the field? In P. McCardle, S. McCune, J. A. Griffin, & V. Maholmes (Eds.), *How animals affect us: Examining the influence of human-animal interaction on child development and human health* (pp. 35-52). Washington, DC: American Psychological Association Press.

Kienzle, E., Bergler, R., & Mandernach, A. (1998) Comparison of the feeding behavior and the human animal relationship in owners of normal and obese dogs. *Journal of Nutrition, 128*, 2779S.

Lumeng, J. C., Forrest, P., Appugliese, D. P., Kaciroti, N., Corwyn, R. F., & Bradley R. H. (2010). Weight status as a predictor of being bullied in third through sixth grades. *Pediatrics, 125*(6), 1301-1307.

Marino, L., & Lilienfeld, S. O. (2007). Dolphin-assisted therapy: More flawed data and more flawed conclusions. *Anthrozoos, 20*(3), 239-249.

McNicholas, J., & Collis, G. (2000). Dogs as catalysts for social interactions: Robustness of the effect. *British Journal of Psychology, 91*(Pt 1), 61-70.

Messent, P. R. (1983). Social facilitation of contact with other people by pet dogs. In A. H. Katcher & A. M. Beck (Eds.), *New perspectives on our lives with companion animals* (pp. 37-46). Philadelphia: University of Pennsylvania Press.

Monterio, P., et al. (2003). Birth size, early childhood growth, and adolescent obesity in a Brazilian birth cohort *International Journal of Obesity, 27*, 1274-1282.

Morris, P. J., Montoya, J. A., Bautista, I., Juste, M. C., Suarez, L., Peña, C., McCune, S., & Hackett, R.M. (2007). The effect of owner weight status on the relationship between owner and dog. Poster presentation at the IAHAIO conference, Tokyo, Japan.

Motooka, M., Koike, H., Yokoyama, T., & Kennedy, N. (2006). Effect of dog-walking on autonomic nervous activity in senior citizens. *Medical Journal of Australia, 184*(2), 60-63.

Ogden, C. L., Carroll, M. D., Curtin, L. R., Lamb, M. M., & Flegal, K. (2010). Prevalence of high body mass index in US children and adolescents, 2007-2008. *Journal of the American Medical Association, 303*, 242-249.

Plachta-Danielzik, S., Landsberg, B., Bosy-Westphal, A., Johannsen, M., Lange, D., & Müller, M. J. (2008). Energy gain and energy gap in normal weight children: Longitudinal data of the KOPS. *Obesity, 16,* 777–783.

Sterl, P., & Brandenburg, C. (2008). Visitors' awareness and assessment of recreational disturbance of wildlife in the Donau-Auen National Park. *Journal for Nature Conservation, 16*(3), 135-145.

Wang, Y. C., Gortmaker, S. L., Sobol, A. M., & Kuntz, K. M. (2006). Estimating the energy gap among US children: A counterfactual approach. *Pediatrics, 118,* 1721-1733.

Index